CF 9.20
1999/1029

Date Due

OCT 1 4 2020		
JUN 2 4 2022		
JUN 0 7 2023		

BRODART, CO.   Cat. No. 23-233   Printed in U.S.A.

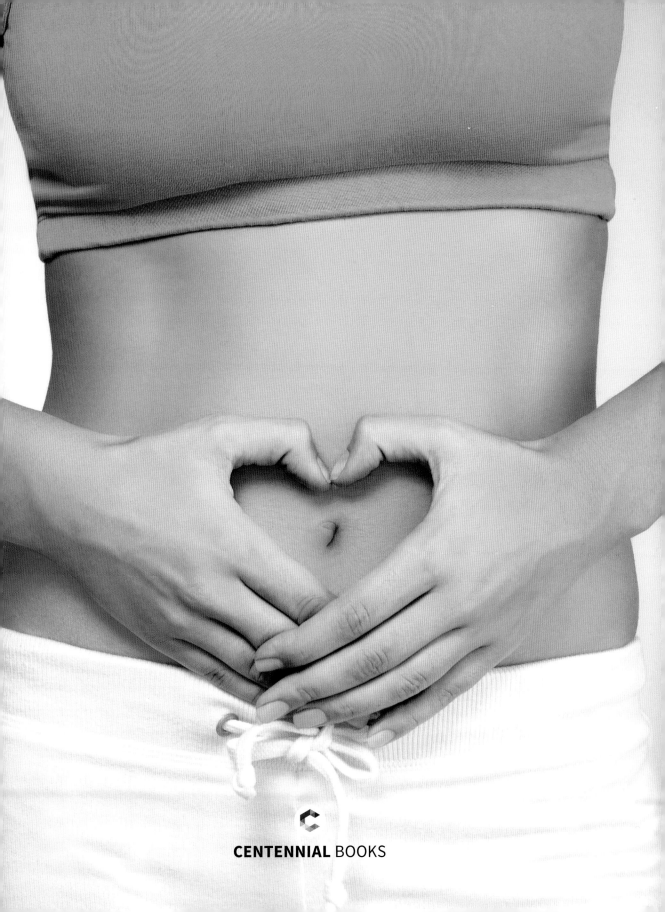

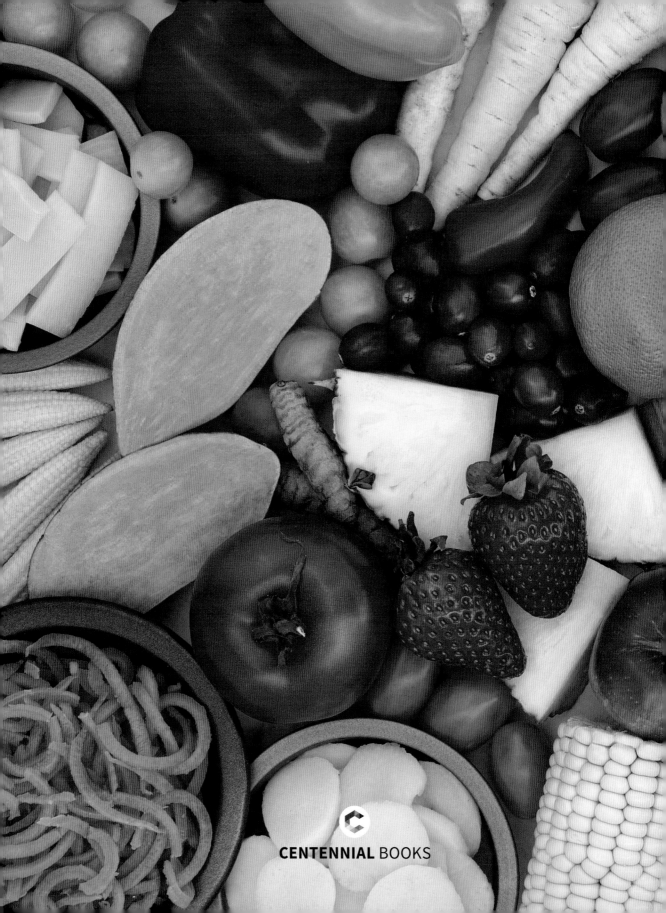

CENTENNIAL BOOKS

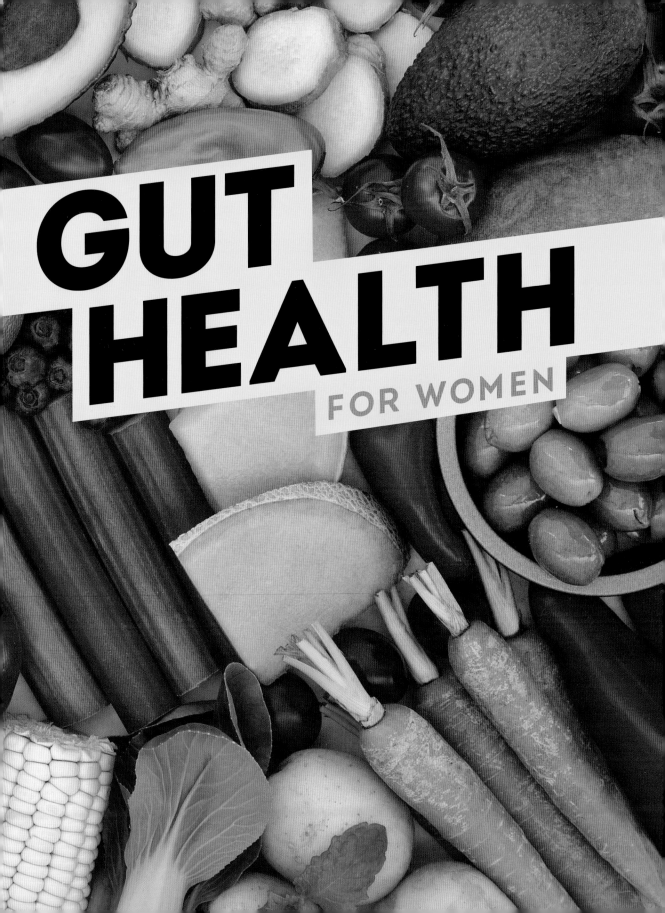

GUT
HEALTH
FOR WOMEN

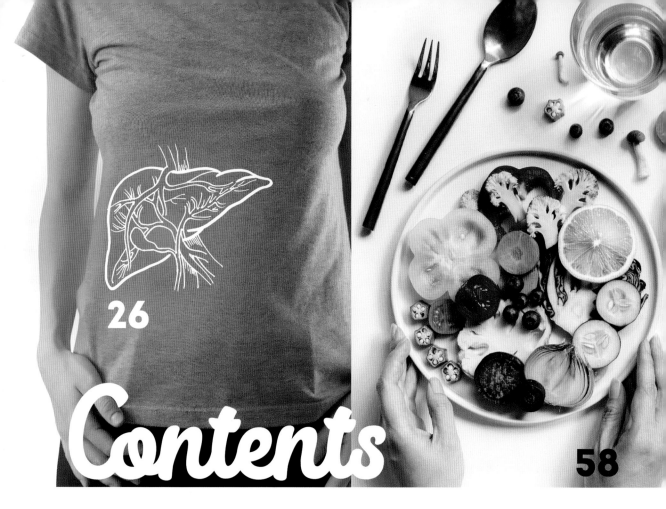

26

58

Contents

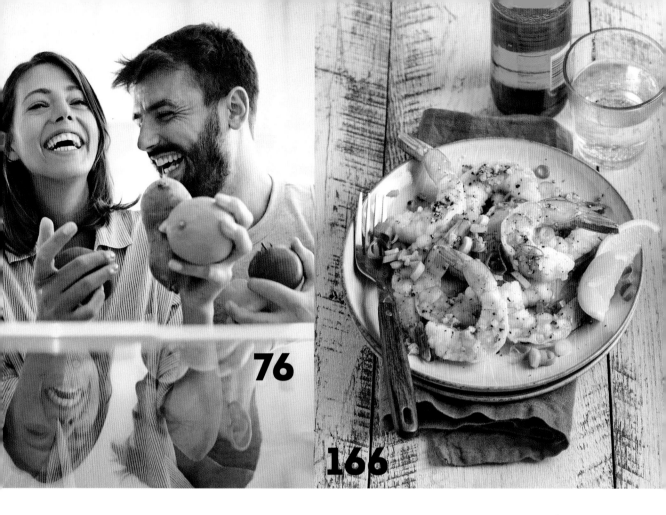

76

166

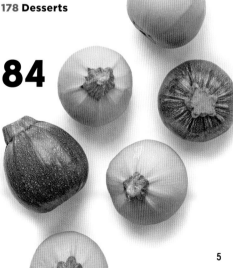

84

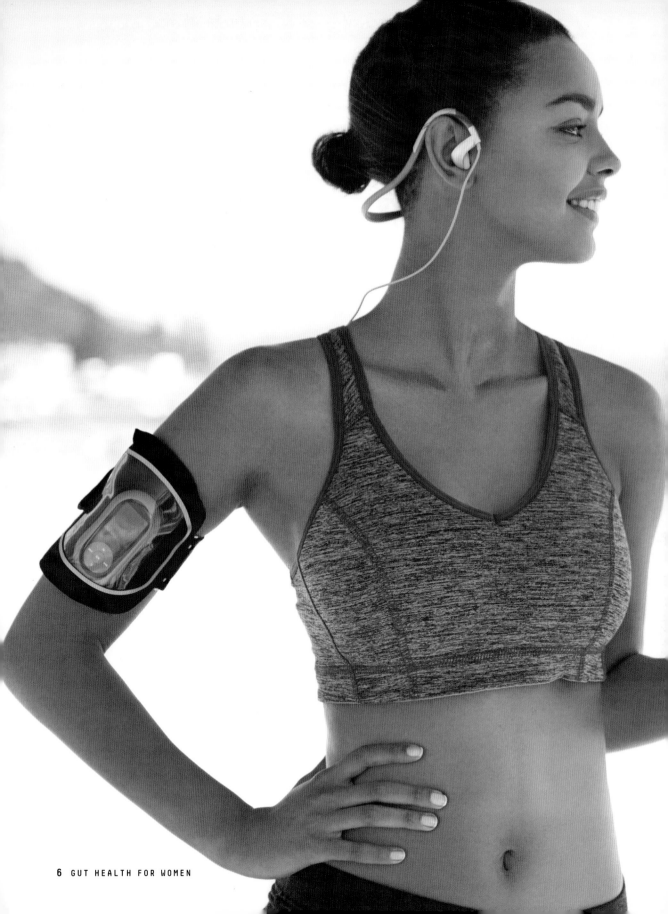

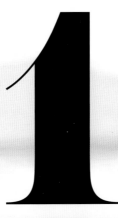

1

The Magic in the Machine

THE DIGESTIVE SYSTEM WORKS IN MANY
WONDERFUL AND MYSTERIOUS WAYS
—AND RESEARCHERS ARE JUST BEGINNING
TO UNDERSTAND WHAT THIS MEANS FOR OUR HEALTH.

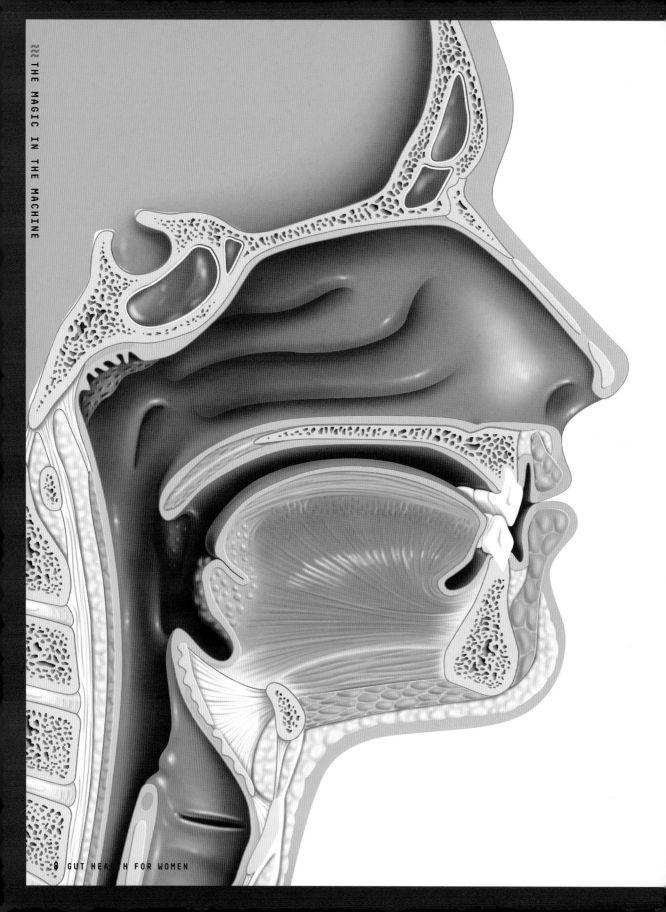

DOWN THE
hatch!

*SO MUCH HAPPENS DURING THE 24 TO 36 HOURS
IT TYPICALLY TAKES FOR FOOD TO MOVE
THROUGH YOUR DIGESTIVE TRACT.*

Digestion may seem pretty straightforward: Food goes in, makes its way through what is essentially a long, hollow tube, and within a day or so it goes out. The system is designed to break down that steak or avocado on your fork into nutrients your body can use. Like a chop shop, whatever you put in gets stripped for parts—carbohydrates, protein and fat; vitamins, minerals and fiber. And yet the process is also incredibly nuanced. Hormonal shifts, stress, allergens, nutrients, circadian rhythms and more can all impact the gut and throw off the process. Feeling chronically stressed? The signals between your brain and bowel may get disrupted, leading to constipation, abdominal pain and more. Sleep-deprived? Key hormones that control hunger may go haywire, prompting you to eat more and gain weight. When communication gets messed up, or the food you're eating isn't good quality or contains things you're sensitive to, that's where the system breaks down.

"There's so much that can go wrong in the gut, and our standard American diet doesn't help," says food scientist Laura Rokosz, PhD, founder of EgglRock Nutrition in New Jersey. "Overly processed foods and even seemingly 'healthy' foods can trigger inflammation in the body." The good news: Cleaning up your diet and lifestyle can lead to amazing and unexpected shifts in your health—and there's plenty of help here.

Turn the page for a look at the intricate gastrointestinal (GI) tract.

IT'S

Alimentary,

MY DEAR

FROM YOUR MOUTH TO YOUR BACKSIDE, HERE'S HOW
YOUR BODY TACKLES THE FOOD YOU GIVE IT EVERY DAY.

Despite taking place in what is essentially a long tube–aka the gastrointestinal (GI) tract or alimentary canal–digestion is a complicated process. There are different stages along the way–kind of like a factory assembly line, except the food is being disassembled and turned into energy, nutrition and waste. If you're eating a healthy diet and living a balanced lifestyle, you may not have to think twice about it. Let's take a peek inside.

1 Like the beginning of a car wash, the chewing process provides the initial rinse. The **TEETH** break up food, and enzymes in the mouth start the initial phase of digestion. You probably don't realize it, but your **MOUTH** is armed with a number of chemical defenses to keep foreign bacteria out. In fact, it's the first line of defense against bad bugs.

2 The enzyme **SALIVARY AMYLASE** is released in the mouth to start the digestion of carbohydrates, which are essentially sugar molecules. The pancreas will later release pancreatic amylase in the small intestine.

Two different types of **SALIVARY GLANDS** (extrinsic and intrinsic) help moisten food and provide enzymes that will later break down carbohydrates and fat. It's a complicated process triggered by receptors in the oral cavity that notify the brain stem and the nervous system.

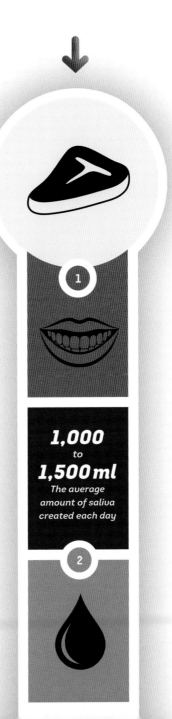

1

1,000
to
1,500 ml
The average amount of saliva created each day

2

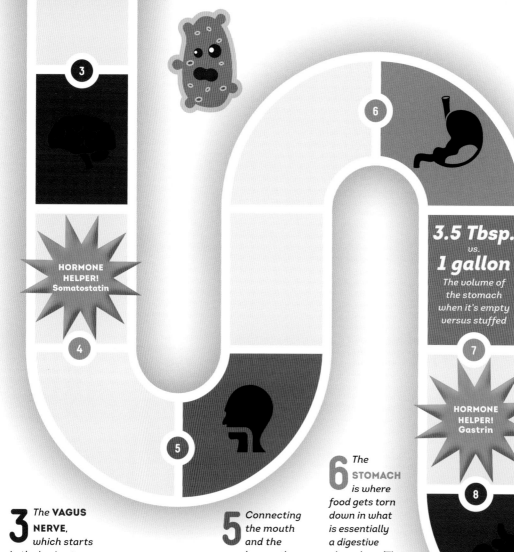

HORMONE HELPER!
Somatostatin

3.5 Tbsp.
vs.
1 gallon
The volume of the stomach when it's empty versus stuffed

HORMONE HELPER!
Gastrin

3 The **VAGUS NERVE**, which starts in the brain stem and "wanders" throughout the body, has a huge role in digestion under the direction of the parasympathetic (rest-and-digest) nervous system. When the sympathetic (fight-or-flight) nervous system kicks in, digestion slows, so resources can be directed elsewhere to address the perceived threat.

4 SOMATOSTATIN is produced in the stomach and small intestine. This hormone slams the brakes on digestion when the sympathetic (fight-or-flight) nervous system sends down signals that there's a fire to put out.

5 Connecting the mouth and the esophagus, the PHARYNX's job is to direct food to move down. Peristalsis, the automatic pushing of food through the system, kicks in at the ESOPHAGUS. It pierces the diaphragm on its way to the stomach. Various sphincters work to keep food in the stomach, but when they fail, that's when you get heartburn.

6 The STOMACH is where food gets torn down in what is essentially a digestive chop shop. (The stomach starts ramping up the digestion process at just the smell, sight or thought of food that appeals to you.) Gastric juice shoots out of pits, carrying hydrochloric acid and pepsin (an enzyme to digest proteins), among other things. Cells in the stomach also secrete intrinsic factor, which allows the body to absorb vitamin B12.

7 GASTRIN stimulates protein digestion in the stomach and the movement of food (now called "chyme") into the small intestine, where nutrient absorption occurs.

Do You Need a Prescription?

Q. HOW CAN I FIND OUT WHICH GUT BUGS I HAVE?

A. The easiest and least invasive way is to test your poop, which you can do in a doctor's office (they'll send it to a lab) or via a mail-in test. Otherwise, you'd have to do a biopsy of the gut, which would be painful and risky. But unless you have some sort of serious disorder going on—or are just curious—it won't do you much good. There's no one "ideal" gut picture and no surefire way to increase or decrease certain bacteria, beyond antibiotics. (The best thing you can do to adjust your gut microbiome is to eat a healthy diet with plenty of fiber, exercise, manage your stress and get plenty of sleep.) If you were to take a peek, you might find the following critters under the microscope:

FAECALIBACTERIUM PRAUSNITZII *One of the most predominant gut bugs, accounting for about 5 percent of the total, F. prausnitzii is in the Firmicute phylum. People with Crohn's disease often have lower numbers of it.*

LACTOBACILLUS *Another common Firmicute, more than a dozen species of lactobacillus populate the gut. Some live there full-time, but others are just traveling through. Research speculates that many arrive there as probiotics in food, including L. acidophilus, L. casei and L. rhamnosus.*

E. COLI *This nasty bug resides in most people without causing an issue; it actually works to defend the intestines from outside invaders, and it makes vitamin K. It's the more virulent strain that you get from contaminated food or water that's the problem.*

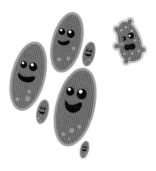

~

CONSTIPATION
Food progresses too slowly through the system, enabling more water to be extracted, which dries out the feces, making it hard to get through.

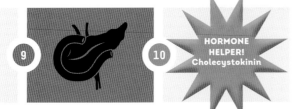

⑨ ⑩

HORMONE HELPER!
Cholecystokinin

8 *The lining of the* **SMALL INTESTINE** *contains microvilli: tiny fingers of tissue that absorb nutrients. Protein, fat and digestible carbs are fully broken down and absorbed in this 20-foot stretch.*

9 *The* **PANCREAS** *secretes its own "juice"— lipase, trypsin, pancreatic amylase and more—into the small intestine to digest nutrients and maintain the pH balance of the blood.*

10 **CHOLECYSTOKININ** *(CCK), a hormone, tells the gallbladder to send some bile to the small intestine to help digest fats. It also triggers the release of pancreatic juice from the pancreas.*

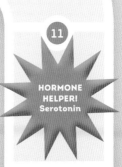

⑪

HORMONE HELPER!
Serotonin

11
SEROTONIN
One of the "feel-good" hormones, which is actually produced in bulk in the gut, it keeps food moving through the intestines (known as motility). Some researchers believe irritable bowel syndrome (IBS) may be related to altered serotonin function in the gut.

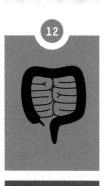

12

100 million

The number of neurons in the enteric nervous system

What's a Biofilm?

Just like animals travel together for protection, groups of microbes often bind together into a plaque or matrix. Think of it as a gooey, sticky netting onto which microbes attach, forming a community. This patch of microbes then sticks to a part of the gut, like putting a big gelatinous bandage across your skin. Good bugs can form a biofilm too, but in the case of bad bugs, their biofilm prevents antibiotics and the body's own immune system from eradicating them. The matrix also enables microbes to communicate easily, like their own bug Facebook group. Although the gut has mechanisms to keep these biofilms from settling in, when there's chronic inflammation—from diet, stress, illness or other lifestyle triggers—the biofilms can overcome your innate defenses. They are common in people who have intestinal disorders, such as inflammatory bowel disease.

13

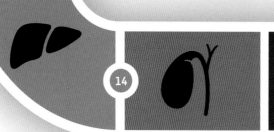

14

500

The number of metabolic functions performed by liver cells, called hepatocytes

12 There's a separate switchboard or "brain" for things that happen in the gut, and it's located within the muscles of the GI tract. Called the **ENTERIC NERVOUS SYSTEM**, it works with the sympathetic and parasympathetic systems, but also calls its own shots.

13 The **LIVER** is a multitasker; it produces bile—which dissolves fats—and sends it to the gallbladder for storage. It also receives blood from the digestive tract and has a role in carb, protein and fat metabolism, plus detoxifying the blood.

14 Tucked up under the liver, the **GALLBLADDER** stores bile and releases it into the first part of the small intestine.

~

DIARRHEA
Food moves too quickly through the large intestine. This prevents water from being re-absorbed, leading to watery stools.

15 Nutrient absorption is mostly done by the time food reaches the **LARGE INTESTINE**, or colon, so named because the tube is much larger here. It travels up the right side of the body, across the middle and down the left before ending in the anal canal.

Layering Up

The walls of the digestive tract are made up of four layers: mucosa, submucosa, muscularis externa and serosa. The construction of these layers diverges slightly, depending on the part of the digestive tract.

The **MUCOSA** absorbs nutrients, secretes hormones and other key players, and wards off invaders, with the help of GALT, gut-associated lymphoid tissue.

The **SUBMUCOSA** allows the stomach and other organs to swell with food and then go back to their original shape.

The **MUSCULARIS EXTERNA** contains two muscle layers, separated by a layer of nerves. It keeps food moving through the system, or temporarily halts it if there's a backup or other issue. In the stomach, the muscularis has an extra layer that helps pummel the food.

The **SEROSA** is the outermost layer and the last level of protection.

15

200 sq. meters
The surface area—used for absorbing nutrients—in the small intestine

500 to 1,000
The number of distinct bacteria species living in the gut

16

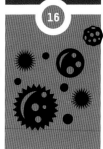

16 The large intestine is populated by trillions of bacteria and other "bugs"—called **MICROBIOTA**. They feed on any remaining undigested food, and their waste products get absorbed by the intestines before the remaining unusable material is pushed out as feces. Researchers are only beginning to understand how important this thriving community is to our health. These bugs are responsible for modulating the immune system as well as creating nutrients, such as vitamin K and short-chain fatty acids, which the large intestine then absorbs, along with water.

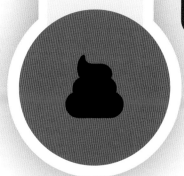

THE
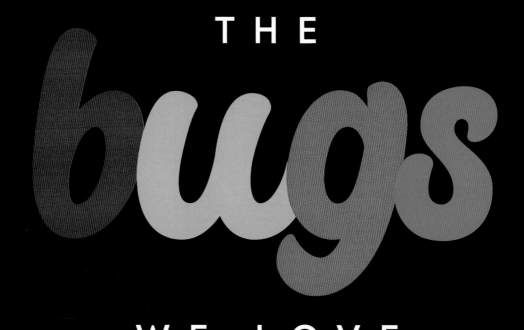
bugs
WE LOVE

*GET TO KNOW THE TINY ORGANISMS
THAT PLAY SUCH AN IMPORTANT ROLE IN YOUR HEALTH.*

To borrow from *Sesame Street*, these are the critters in your neighborhood...specifically, the 5-foot-long section of large intestine called the colon. There's about 100 trillion—up to 4 pounds of them—in the average adult gut; these single-celled organisms are diverse, but only a handful dominate. Their main function is to consume certain types of carbohydrates and other nutrients that make their way through the gut. That process results in short-chain fatty acids (acetate, butyrate and propionate—sometimes called post-biotics) that your body uses for fuel and other important functions. They also help keep pathogenic invaders (and residents) in check, and maintain the immune system and gut lining. The state of your microbe population has been linked with all sorts of health problems outside the gut, including heart disease, cancer, asthma and eczema.

PROTEOBACTERIA
These proliferate in certain inflammatory conditions such as type 2 diabetes, obesity, asthma, bowel disorders and cardiovascular disease. Shigella, Rickettsia, Bordetella, Salmonella, Helicobacter and E. coli are all proteobacteria.

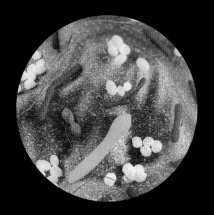

FIRMICUTES

These bacteria include lactobacillus, streptococcus, mycoplasma and clostridium. Firmicutes, along with bacteroidetes, dominate the colon. They gobble up carbs and excrete short-chain fatty acids, which nourish the cells lining the gut and turn into energy.

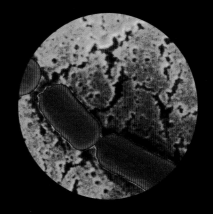

BACTEROIDETES

Responsible for nasty infections if they escape the intestines, these bacteria are benign when they're just in the colon. True sugar specialists, bacteroidetes feast on carbs. They also play a role in the gut's immune system as well as other immune responses.

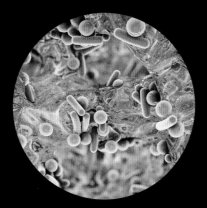

ACTINOBACTERIA

The most famous genus here is bifidobacterium, a common probiotic found in yogurt. Shifts in bifidobacterium levels are often involved in dysbiosis—a change in the balance of gut bugs that's often associated with a host of diseases.

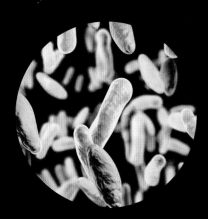

CANDIDA

Different types of this fungus (particularly C. albicans) can cause vaginal yeast and serious fungal infections—but it's commonly found in the intestinal tract. The surrounding good bacteria keep candida in check. Vegetarians tend to have lower levels of candida.

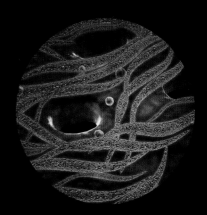

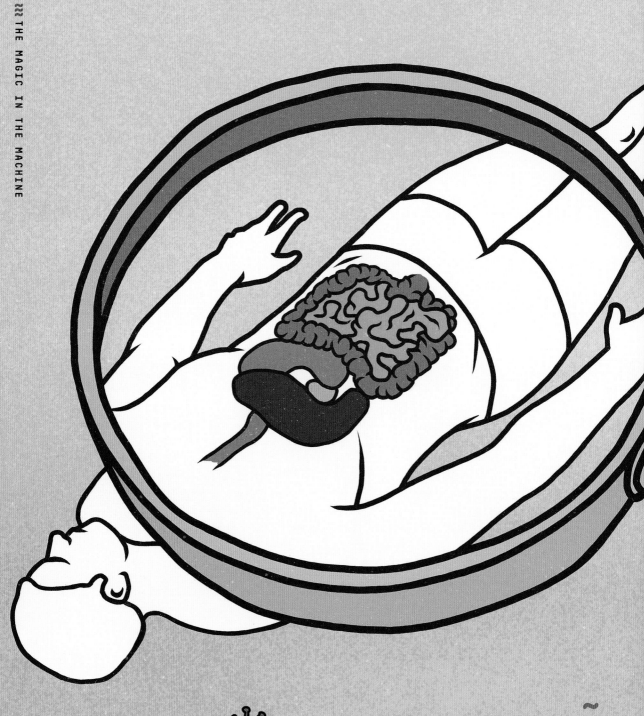

Your belly
is a big bug
wonderland.

Gut Stuff

THIS NEW FRONTIER IN MEDICINE AND HEALTH WILL CHANGE EVERYTHING.

You can't read health headlines these days without seeing something about the gut microbiome and gut health. Scientists continue to link it to aspects of both our physical and mental health, so much so that many experts proclaim: "It all starts with the gut." And that's not an overstatement.

"A healthy gut microbiota leads to a healthy body," says Justin Sonnenburg, PhD, an associate professor of microbiology and immunology at Stanford University. "Actually, it starts with a healthy diet. We make decisions about what we eat, so we hold the control to nurture the gut microbes that affect our mood, behavior, immune system, metabolism and beyond."

But this association is much more complex than many make it seem, he adds. While there have been huge strides in microbiome research in the past decade, there are still so many things yet to be discovered.

Researching the Gut

Many falsely credit Nobel laureate and microbiologist Joshua Lederberg, PhD, for coining the term "microbiome" in 2001. The truth is, other researchers had used the word for years before Lederberg did, and centuries before all of this, scientists began to lay the groundwork for the modern field of microbiology.

But 2001 was a big year for the microbiome, which Lederberg defined as "the ecological community of commensal, symbiotic and pathogenic microorganisms that literally share our body space and have been all but ignored as determinants of health and disease." In that same year, the Human Genome Project—an international group of hundreds of researchers—published a first draft of the human genome sequence.

Since then, the research and interest in gut health have exploded. "The community of microbes in the gut had been ignored for a long period of time because it's complex and difficult to study, and its importance to our health wasn't fully appreciated," Sonnenburg

33

Number of U.S. universities, research institutions and medical schools that have formed microbiome centers

explains. "In the past 10 to 15 years, this field took off. We started by studying what is intuitive—such as how microbes are important in how we digest food and how they impact gut mucosal health—and now we are working to understand more complex interactions between our gut microbes and overall health. We're really making great progress in understanding everything that they do."

This is in part due to organizations like the International Human Microbiome Consortium (IHMC), which launched in 2008. Composed of research organizations from 11 countries, the IHMC aims to prevent and treat diseases by sharing findings on the human microbiome.

Another key factor in the field's growth has been advances in technology. "The first round of data on the human gut microbiome gave us a glimpse of what a healthy microbiome should look like and, when people have diseases, what dysbiosis, or a disrupted microbiome, looks like," explains Liping Zhao, PhD, director of the Center for Nutrition, Microbiome, and Health at Rutgers, the State University of New Jersey. "Now that the field has generated enough data and we have thousands of papers on this, we start to understand what kind of disruption happens to the gut microbiome when a person has a disease like obesity, diabetes, cancer or dementia."

What Goes Around

The link between gut health and these various diseases is still being parsed out by scientists. We know that although bacteria can colonize the entire gastrointestinal tract, the major players are the microbes at the far reaches of the digestive tract, in the colon, Sonnenburg says.

Gut health is linked with more than 50 diseases.

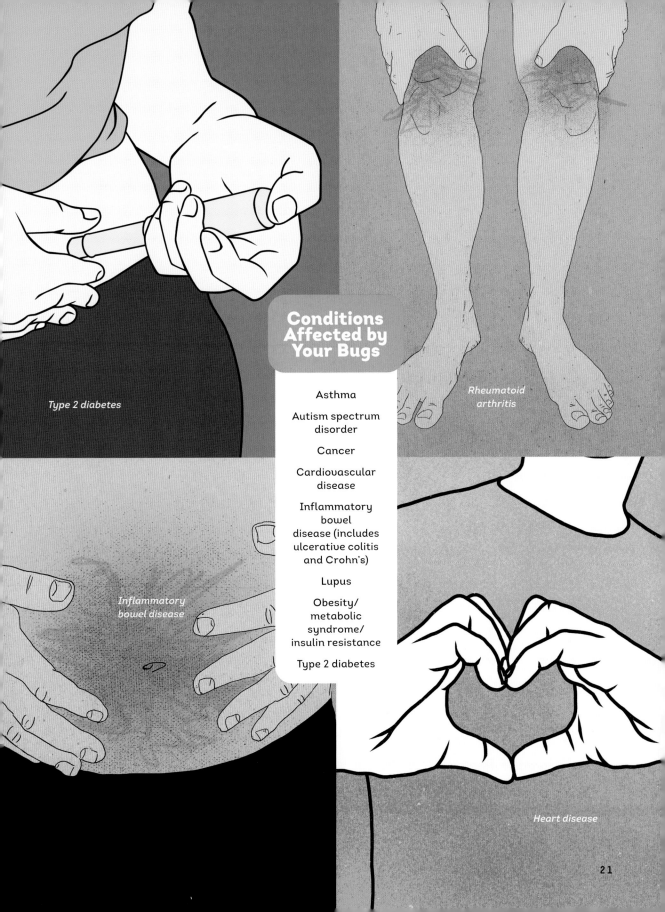

Type 2 diabetes

Rheumatoid arthritis

Inflammatory bowel disease

Conditions Affected by Your Bugs

Asthma

Autism spectrum disorder

Cancer

Cardiovascular disease

Inflammatory bowel disease (includes ulcerative colitis and Crohn's)

Lupus

Obesity/ metabolic syndrome/ insulin resistance

Type 2 diabetes

Heart disease

"The lower gut is a perfect paradise for microorganisms," says Zhao. "It has a consistent supply of various nutrients, the temperature is constant, and the pH is no longer too acidic—they're almost the perfect conditions to allow bacteria and other microorganisms to grow." When these microbes ferment prebiotics (essentially, fiber that passes through the first part of the GI system mostly untouched), they produce various bioactive compounds. Some, such as short-chain fatty acids, are essential to health. Others can be detrimental, such as toxins that can stimulate inflammation, induce cancers or drive neurodegenerative disease or autism, Zhao explains.

The effects of these compounds seem to be bidirectional: Changes in the gut can modulate various systems throughout the body, and those systems can also regulate the gut environment.

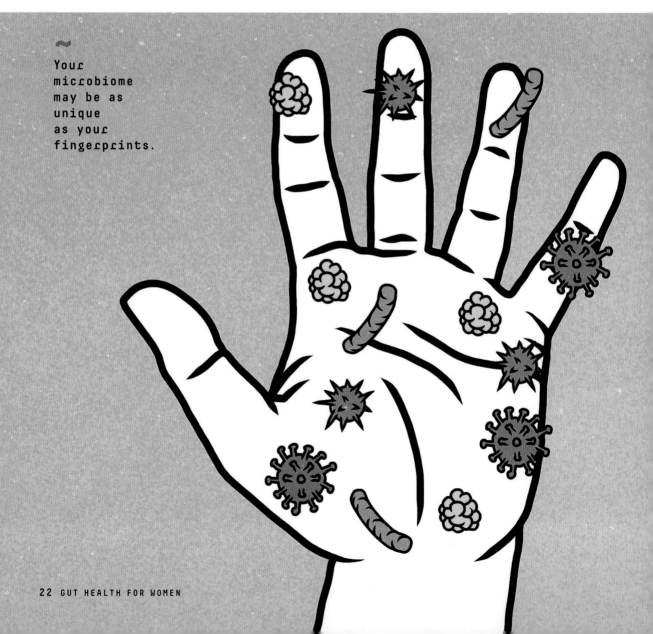

Your microbiome may be as unique as your fingerprints.

"Our body is this big integrative system. All of these parts are talking to other parts," Sonnenburg says. "If you incite inflammation, the immune response can change the gut microbiota and dictate what microbes are there. In return, these microbes can send signals to change other aspects of physiology."

Researchers have established potential links between changes in the gut microbiota and the development of more than 50 kinds of diseases, Zhao says. These include type 2 diabetes, cancer, skin diseases, cardiovascular diseases and inflammatory bowel disease. And more and more evidence is emerging. "Different people may have different bacteria overgrowing and different symptoms [of a condition], but rigorous scientific data supports the hypothesis that the gut is the primary source of the disease-driving molecules produced by overgrowing pathogenic bacteria," he says.

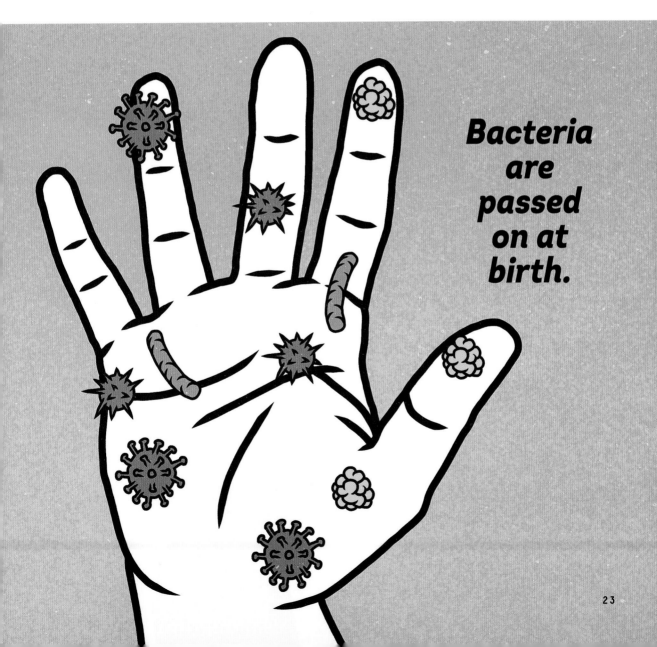

Bacteria are passed on at birth.

The Future Looks Bright

While all of this is exciting, there's also some reason to be cautious. "From the scientific perspective, gut health is still not emphasized enough. But whether we can use this new knowledge to teach people how to improve their gut health, the application and translational side of this development is still too early," Zhao says.

Both he and Sonnenburg caution against companies that promise to tell you all about your gut and overall health from one fecal sample. "The science is not mature enough to support such direct implication to consumers," Zhao stresses. New, more powerful technology to sequence different strains of bacteria and mine the data is needed to bring the science to the clinical level and actually help people, he adds. The reason: No one bacterial strain is shared by everybody—at most, one strain may show up in no more than 5 percent of the population. "The database [on a global level] is very limited," says Zhao.

However, many new developments are in the works to overcome these hurdles. "This will revolutionize almost everything related to health—the food industry, pharma, health care—it's disrupting everything," Zhao says. "But it may take 10 to 20 years, and we need to be cautious when educating the general public about the findings."

For now, we know that the best way to foster a healthy gut is to limit the amount of antibiotics you take and eat a diet rich in fibers from foods such as legumes, whole grains, vegetables, fruits and nuts, Sonnenburg says. "If you're eating a typical Western diet [full of sugars and processed foods], your microbes will start to eat the mucus lining of the gut, and that can lead to inflammation and negative health consequences."

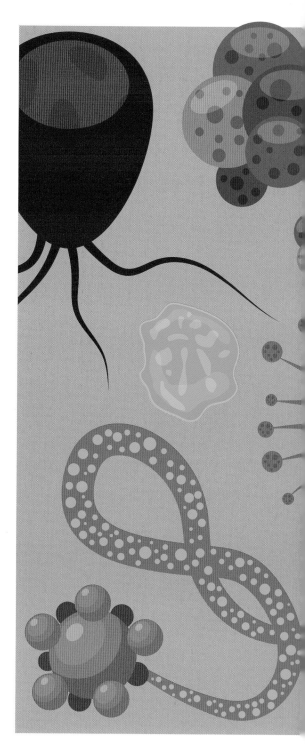

Don't Panic About Parasites

The word "parasite" is enough to give many people the creepy-crawlies, but according to some alternative- and functional-medicine doctors, almost everyone has them. Don't freak out just yet about these freeloaders, though.

"Not everyone is riddled with parasites, but they are more common than we thought," says naturopathic medicine doctor Kara Fitzgerald, ND, director of The Sandy Hook Clinic in Newtown, Connecticut.

First, where you live matters. "In areas of the U.S. where parasites are regularly seen [such as the Gulf Coast], it is possible that people may harbor them without knowing, since some present without any symptoms or with very mild symptoms," adds Bernard JC Macatangay, MD, an infectious-disease physician at the University of Pittsburgh Medical Center. "In other areas where parasites aren't common or regularly seen, it's less likely for people to have them," unless they've recently traveled.

Most people acquire parasites through eating contaminated food or drinking contaminated water, being bitten by a mosquito or other insect, ingesting or coming into contact with contaminated soil, through sexual transmission, or through transmission from an infected mother to her baby during childbirth.

Although you can find all sorts of remedies online, medication is usually the best way to get rid of the little bugs. Botanicals such as wormwood and black walnut may help, but these can also be harsh on the liver, so only use them under the direction of a trained physician, says Fitzgerald.

Some parasites will die on their own, but others can live for several years, Macatangay says. The best treatment depends on which parasite you have, which is why a proper diagnosis is key. An infectious-disease doctor can run tests. "It's not cost-effective to test for them if there has been no travel to areas where parasites are common," Macatangay adds.

Your doctor may test your stool, blood, vaginal fluid, urine or skin, Fitzgerald says. From there, she'll discuss the proper treatment to kill the critters and explain how to best avoid them in the future.

Disease can
stem from
a slow burn.

THE FIRE IN YOUR
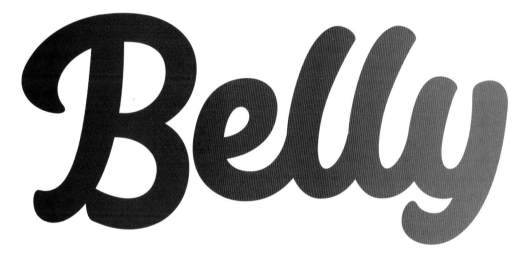

AS RESEARCHERS DIG FURTHER INTO THE POWER OF THE MICROBIOME, THEY ARE UNCOVERING ITS INFLUENCE OVER THE IMMUNE SYSTEM AND THE ROLE IT PLAYS IN SYSTEMIC HEALTH ISSUES.

Inflammation is a word that we've been hearing more and more of lately. It used to bring to mind the swelling that would occur if you sprained your ankle, broke your arm or had a tooth infection, but now it's considered a culprit in heart disease, obesity, some cancers and even autoimmune diseases, not to mention seemingly benign health issues such as eczema, fatigue, weight gain (or loss) and joint pain.

Inflammation can be a lot more subtle (and dangerous) than a ballooned-up ankle—there's more to it than meets the eye—but the root cause of it hasn't always been clear. Acute inflammation is the body's short-term response to injury. In the case of that swollen ankle, it's your immune system going to bat for you, initiating healing. Something similar happens in the digestive tract (see page 8) where the bugs have to fend off pathogens like viruses, bacteria, parasites or fungi, and even environmental pollutants and chemicals. As the backbone of the immune system, the microbiome is constantly mounting an inflammatory response to fend off invaders. How well the gut can do this is the difference between a healthy immune system and a weak one that's vulnerable to chronic inflammation and more.

"What people don't realize is that the gut, in a sense, is outside of the body," says Lynn Wagner, MD, who runs an integrative-medicine practice at BayCare Clinic in De Pere, Wisconsin. The digestive tract is a hollow lumen, or cavity, running through the body, and its walls separate it from the organs, muscles and fluids of the body. It functions like a waiting room for anything coming in from the outside—a place to vet new arrivals and keep intruders from moving to the inner rooms. "It constantly works to protect our internal environment from what's coming in," says Wagner.

TIP
Allergy testing isn't foolproof, so always work with a doc.

Lining the lumen of the digestive tract is the gut-associated lymphoid tissue (GALT). It's permeable, since it assists with food absorption, but it also works overtime to fend off antigens and perceived invaders.

"There are more immune-system cells in our gut and more cells in the microbiome than there are in rest of the entire body," Wagner says. "And so, the immune system is in large part the GALT." It's like a gatekeeper to the bloodstream and the rest of the body, so it's easy to see how inflammation can get a foothold.

Tipping the Balance

"There are trillions of cells inside the gut —bacteria, viruses, fungi and potentially parasites—a bunch of different types of bugs. They all have different functions and all of them can turn into a problem if they become too dominant. It's a delicate balance," Wagner adds.

Aided by the GALT, a healthy gut will recognize a pathogen and mount an immune response to attack it and get rid of it, says Wagner. If there's an imbalance in the microbiome, it becomes easier for the bad bugs to get a foothold. Antibiotics, infections, food sensitivities, bacteria in food, a poor diet, even trauma and stress, can all alter the microbiome.

Leaky gut is another culprit in inflammation. "The lining of the gut, which includes the GALT, is one cell layer thick. Each cell is tightly bound to the one next to it. These cells have villi facing into the gut, which decide what stays in the lumen or digestive tract and what can go into the body," explains Wagner. Leaky gut occurs when the junctures holding the cells together loosen or start to pull apart, allowing small particles to escape through the lining, triggering an immune response. However intrusive particles are making it through the gut barrier, if they're constantly getting through the gut wall, then

"The GALT decides if it has to mount an immune response to keep things out."

Lynn Wagner, MD

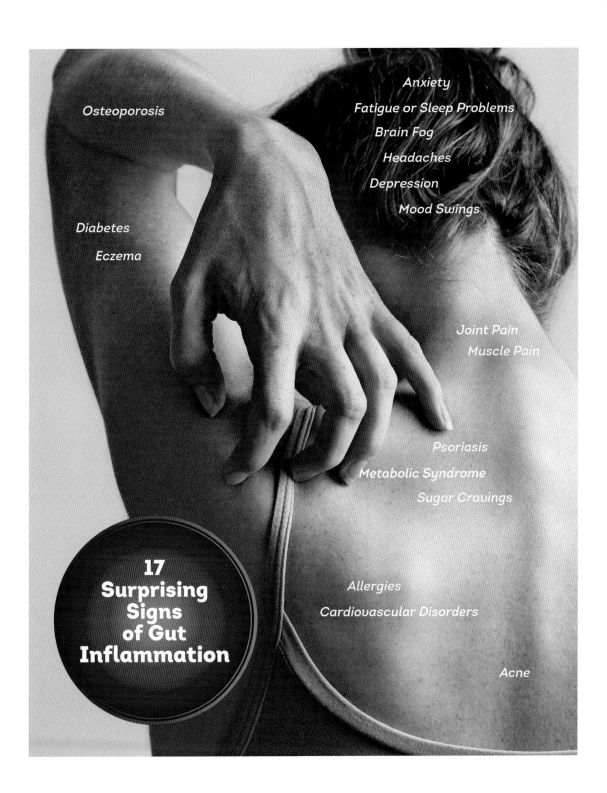

Osteoporosis

Anxiety

Fatigue or Sleep Problems

Brain Fog

Headaches

Depression

Mood Swings

Diabetes

Eczema

Joint Pain

Muscle Pain

Psoriasis

Metabolic Syndrome

Sugar Cravings

17 Surprising Signs of Gut Inflammation

Allergies

Cardiovascular Disorders

Acne

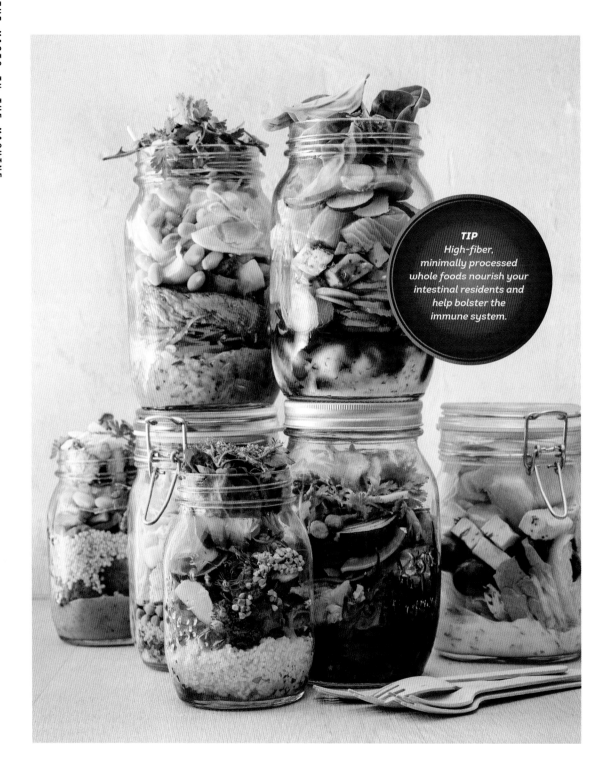

TIP
High-fiber, minimally processed whole foods nourish your intestinal residents and help bolster the immune system.

the immune response is constantly triggered and inflammation becomes chronic. The many different ways the microbiome can be disrupted is why Wagner says, "When people have issues with autoimmune disease, chronic pain, obesity or mental health, I always start with the gut."

The (Not So) Missing Link

Now that researchers around the world are focusing more on the microbiome, there seems to be no shortage of scientific findings to support how a disruption to it has an adverse effect on our overall health. In a 2019 study published in *The Journal of Physiology*, researchers found that changes in the microbiome over time can have a harmful impact on vascular health. The study, which was done on mice, provided the "first evidence for the gut microbiome being an important mediator of age-related arterial dysfunction and oxidative stress," said the authors.

Rogue bugs escaping the GI tract can upend the whole system.

Although it has been established that oxidative stress and inflammation can have a negative impact on arterial health over time, researchers have not previously been able to pinpoint what causes arteries to become inflamed and stressed. In the study, the researchers saw an increased prevalence of pro-inflammatory microbes that are associated with disease in older mice. These findings, the authors say, open up future opportunities for targeted therapies and interventions to prevent cardiovascular disease.

Similarly, another new study, also with mice and published in *Cancer Research*, found that a compromised microbiome resulted in

Foods That Promote Inflammation

Instead of heading to the doctor to see what's wrong with you, try opening your kitchen cabinets first. According to author Raphael Kellman, MD, foods that alter the microbiome and trigger inflammation include sugar and other processed or artificial sweeteners (some, such as stevia, are referred to as "natural" even though they are processed); sugar-sweetened beverages; processed grains, including any product made with white flour; gluten-bearing grains, including wheat, barley and rye, which are also added to many foods, including condiments; cow's milk and dairy; eggs; soy; red meat and processed meats, such as hot dogs, sausage and bacon; and foods made with artificial ingredients such as preservatives and dyes. Many of these are also common food allergens, which the body identifies as harmful.

"You have to cut out anything highly processed, anything that is high in sugar," says integrative physician Lynn Wagner, MD. "Get the bad or unhealthy fats out." While you're at it, cut out (or cut back on) alcohol and ditch the smoking habit. Simply reducing your intake of these types of foods and substances may spur a change in how you feel, eliminating the need for pricey tests and drugs.

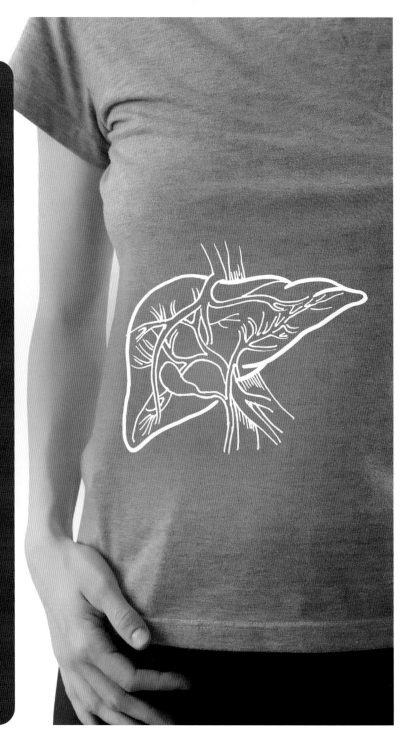

The Gut-Liver Axis

The liver contributes bile to the digestion process, but what happens farther down the GI tract can have adverse effects on this multitasking organ. Numerous studies have linked errant microbes and general gut dysbiosis—too many of the wrong kinds of bugs—to liver diseases, including alcoholic steatohepatitis, portal hypertension, cirrhosis, and nonalcoholic fatty liver disease (NAFLD). Large-scale reviews have estimated a quarter to a third of all U.S. adults have NAFLD. According to the American Liver Foundation, 100 million people have it, and rates in children have doubled in the past two decades. A 2019 review in the journal Diseases *found that probiotics may be able to help reverse dysbiosis and improve liver inflammation and function. More research is still needed, but it's an example of how impacting the microbiome can directly affect another organ.*

inflammation within the mammary tissue and influenced the spread of breast cancer.

A 2017 review of the clinical evidence supporting the microbiome as an important mechanism in the onset and maintenance of inflammation found that "microorganisms are crucial in maintaining gastrointestinal homeostasis and can potently modulate systemic immunity." The researchers noted that while progress is being made in understanding the microbiome's role in inflammatory diseases, more clinical research is needed to find targeted treatments.

What experts do know is that once inflammation gains traction, it can be hard to reduce it and get the immune system back on track unless you heal the gut. "Improving the microbiome, healing the trillions of gut bacteria, is your greatest ally," says Raphael Kellman, MD, founder of the Kellman Center in New York City and author of *The Microbiome Breakthrough* and *The Microbiome Diet*. Chronic fatigue, fibromyalgia, metabolic disturbances such as diabetes, and autoimmune disorders are all linked to inflammation, Kellman says, and too often the medical profession has tried to treat those diseases without acknowledging the role of the microbiome.

Feed Your Gut

Probiotics are a key step to treating the microbiome, with a caveat. "There are different ones for different health issues. You have to know which is the best probiotic for you, based on what's going on. Lactobacillus rhamnosus may be used for anxiety and Lactobacillus reuteri for autoimmune issues. It's very complex," says Kellman. Plus, it's individualized to each patient. Still, there is a baseline approach that can help promote a healthy microbiome, and it involves probiotics and prebiotics. "Prebiotics are a nondigestible fiber found in food such as jicama, artichokes, carrots and radishes that help to nourish the microbiome," he explains. "Fermented foods, aka probiotics, include kimchi, sauerkraut and unflavored yogurt or kefir. They're rich in friendly bacteria like the kind found in the gut."

Eating a "clean" diet and eschewing inflammatory foods can help nourish a healthy digestive (and immune) system, says Wagner. She suggests a diet rich in low-sugar fruits (such as berries, watermelon, kiwis and grapefruit); nuts, seeds and wild salmon that are high in anti-inflammatory omega 3s; and spices, such as turmeric, which acts as a potent anti-inflammatory.

Gut Health and PCOS

Polycystic ovary syndrome (PCOS) is a metabolic and endocrine disorder that affects up to a quarter of women during their reproductive years. Besides having difficulty conceiving, many also show signs of metabolic syndrome, including high blood sugar, cholesterol and blood pressure, and excess weight. A 2017 study published in Frontiers in Microbiology found that women with PCOS, regardless of weight, had the least diverse microbiomes (compared to controls). Women with PCOS had similar dysbiosis of gut microbiota as those who had obesity, and those who had both had the most serious dysbiosis. They also had higher levels of gram-negative bacteria, linked with inflammation and insulin resistance.

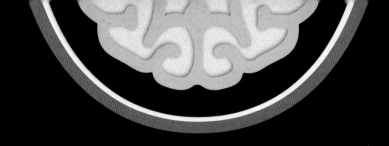

"Hello, Brain? Gut Speaking..."

THERE'S A COMPLEX RELATIONSHIP BETWEEN
OUR TWO BRAINS, AND AS IT TURNS OUT,
THE GUT HAS A LOT TO SAY

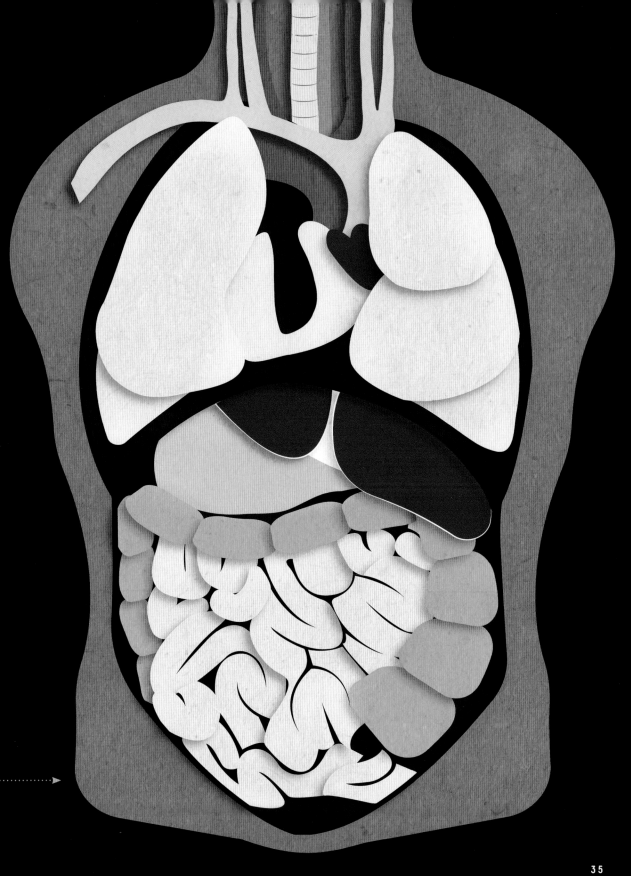

Scientists have known about the "gut-brain connection" for decades, but it hasn't been until recently that studies of the microbiome have started to unveil the significance of this relationship.

"Intuitively, we have known for years that our brain and gut are connected," says Judith Scheman, PhD, director of behavioral medicine for the Digestive Disease and Surgery Institute of the Cleveland Clinic. "It's reflected in our language in the way we describe our emotions." We say things like, "It's gut-wrenching," "That makes me sick" or "I have butterflies in my stomach."

The reason we use those terms is that a number of neurotransmitters (the signals that enable the nervous system to function and communicate) are produced in the gut: As much as 80 to 90 percent of the body's serotonin is synthesized there, as well as 50 percent of the dopamine. "Basically, the action is taking place in our gut, but our brain has a much better vocabulary so it puts words to what's happening farther south," says Scheman.

TIP
Depressed? Try adjusting your diet first.

"We've referred to this relationship forever... and it was really almost dismissed because we thought it wasn't that important—when, in fact, the enteric nervous system [in the digestive tract] is much more complex than it was ever given credit to be," explains Jay Pasricha, MD, director of the Johns Hopkins Center for Neurogastroenterology. "It's highly sophisticated and organized in ways we are just beginning to understand."

The Second Brain—or Is It?

"The gut has its own brain—the enteric nervous system, which is in the walls of the gut," says Pasricha. It consists of hundreds of millions of neurons—more than in the spinal cord— running inside the digestive tract from the esophagus to the rectum. "It consists of layers and layers of nerve cells that can work relatively independently even if they were cut off from the other nervous systems," he says. "In some ways, if you look at evolution, then this is the first brain. This was the first nervous system to form and it's not hard to imagine why. The gut is so critical for its ability to transform energy, in some unusable form, from the environment to something the body can use."

Having a way to monitor and regulate the body is critical to life in higher forms, says Pasricha. "As you go up the food chain, humans are using more complex forms of energy from the environment and you therefore need a system to digest it and for it to work smoothly in the most optimal way. You need a command and control center, and that is where the enteric nerve system is very sophisticated."

That command and control center includes the signals being sent out by the microbiome through the nervous system as it's sensing what's going on in the gut. "Nerves can pick up any signal in the environment. That's their

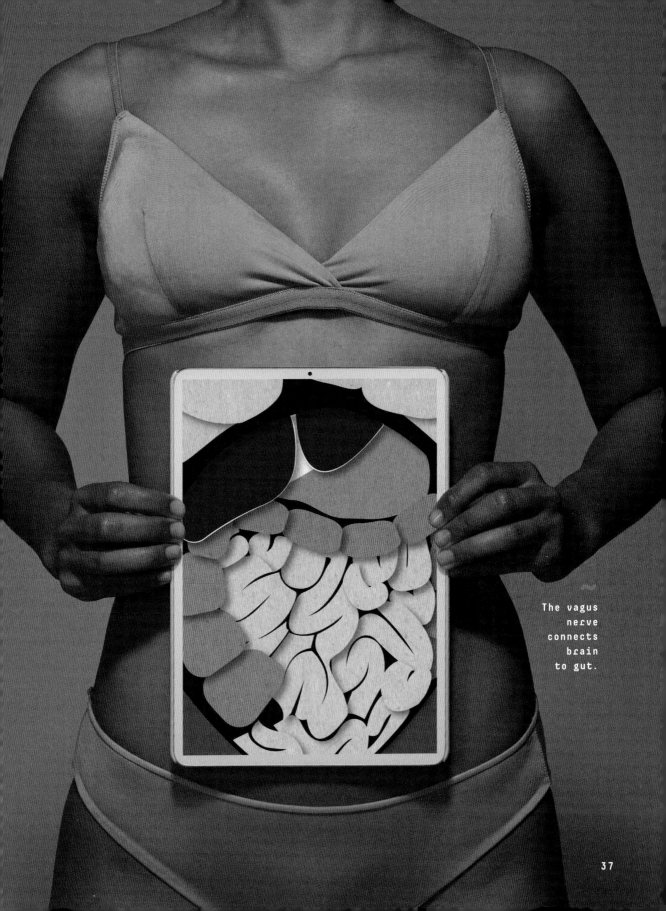

The vagus
nerve
connects
brain
to gut.

job: to relay to headquarters that everything is good—or wait, we have a barbarian at the gate. Raise the alarm! Because of that, the brain and the rest of the body are exquisitely sensitive to signals from these microbes," says Pasricha.

A Three-Way Street

The vagus nerve—aka the 10th cranial nerve, which runs from the brain stem to the colon— is a connector between the gut and the brain. Thanks to it, communication between the gut and the brain goes both ways. "Roughly 90 percent of the communication is going gut to brain and 10 percent from brain to gut," explains Scheman. Neurotransmitters like serotonin play a role in regulating the state of the gut-brain axis, while the microbiome contributes to the effect pathogens have on it.

"The vagus is one of the most important ways to communicate signals from the gut to the brain. Experimental studies show that the vagus nerve is potentially responsible for inducing anxiety and depression in response to gut sensations," Pasricha says. He recounts a study where a mild irritant was used to irritate the colon in baby mice. "When the mice grew up, the ones that had the irritation as pups showed signs of depression and anxiety. There is evidence to suggests the same thing applies to humans."

A more recent study conducted in Europe with two large groups of adults found that certain types of gut bacteria are missing in people with depression. While researchers don't fully understand how an alteration in bacteria can lead to depression, they noted that one of the strains of bacteria missing in the microbiome of depressed participants is associated with dopamine, a neurotransmitter associated with depression. The study also suggested that the vagus nerve is the pathway that carries the awareness of a compromised microbiome to the brain.

What researchers are starting to unravel is that there are many factors that can influence the microbiome and the relationship between the brain and the gut, and also the immune system. While some people are not affected by stress, for those who are it often shows up in the gut (IBS is considered a gut-brain disorder). New research conducted on mice and published in *American Society for Microbiology* showed how chronic social stress altered the composition of the microbiome in a manner that induced a self-destructive change in the immune system. The mice that were exposed to stress were found to have a different microbiome composition, including two particular strains of bacteria that have been linked to autoimmune disorders in humans.

"If the microbiome is disturbed in animals, it can influence the integrity of the central nervous system and the development of the immune system," says Eamonn Quigley, MD, a specialist in gastrointestinal motility disorders and chief of the Division of Gastroenterology and Hepatology at Houston Methodist Hospital. "Having a healthy microbiome can make the gut's reaction to stress less severe—and it's also important for maintaining a good immune system."

"One of the important concepts from research is that our microbiome develops very rapidly from birth to 2 or 3 years of age," says Quigley. Anything—the use of antibiotics, dietary changes, as well as trauma or abuse—that disrupts the microbiome in those first years could have serious long-term consequences. Trauma associated with a life event and chronic stress can each leave a lasting impression on the gut and the microbiome at any stage in life. "We have known for years that trauma makes

TIP
Aim to eat 25 grams of fiber (38 for men) a day.

everything worse and sensitizes the nervous system. The volume gets turned up," says Scheman.

The More We Know, the Less We Know

Add into the mix genetics or environmental factors, and the relationship between the gut and brain gets more complicated. Although experts can see visible changes in the microbiome caused by chronic stress or that indicate depression, they still don't know specifically how these changes came about or if they can be altered. "It is a new and exciting area. There are suggestions, but we need more studies," explains Quigley.

And there lies the crux of the gut-brain connection. The initial hoopla that accompanied the launch of the Human Microbiome Project in 2008 led people to believe health problems could easily be fixed with probiotics and that customized medicine

TIP
Meditation stimulates the vagus nerve, helping calm stress signals.

centered around the microbiome would soon be here. Now, more than a decade later, if there's one thing that's certain, say experts, it's that the more they know, the less they know.

Adding to the complexity is the fact that most of the research conducted on the microbiome is done on mice for now. For ethical reasons, it's difficult to conduct these studies on humans.

While it is clear that a healthy diet and lifestyle can positively affect both overall health and the microbiome, the consensus among experts seems to be that we can see what causes damage, but understanding how to fix the microbiome or heal the gut to fend off disease or mood disorders or enhance cognitive health is a whole other challenge. "It is not simple; there is no magic bullet. Anyone who says they have it figured out, they don't," says Pasricha. "But the benefits of eating a reasonably healthy diet still stand true."

The Mental Health Food Pyramid

You've heard of the food pyramid, and maybe the inflammatory-diet pyramid. Now there's the mental health pyramid. The gut's balance of good and bad bacteria, the GI tract's functioning and the brain's health are all heavily influenced by what you eat and drink. Plan your meals around this pyramid, to help maximize your brain and gut well-being, suggests San Diego naturopathic doctor Heather Tynan, ND.

processed foods sparingly/ avoid!

Red Wine, Dark Chocolate (1–3 servings/ week)

Whole Grains (1–3 servings/day)

Unsaturated Fats (2–4 servings/day)

Lean Protein (2–3 servings/day)

Herbs, Spices and Teas (2–4 servings/day)

Fruits (2–3 servings/day)

Vegetables (6–8 servings/day)

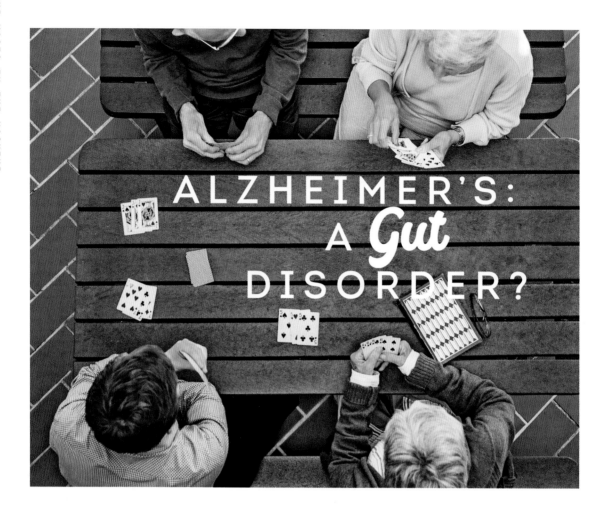

ALZHEIMER'S: A *Gut* DISORDER?

As of 2019, it's estimated that approximately 5.8 million Americans have been diagnosed with Alzheimer's disease. This includes not only the 5.6 million seniors (65 or older) who exhibit symptoms like memory loss, changes in mood or personality, difficulty speaking or writing and confusion about time and place, but also around 200,000 people younger than age 65. Approximately two-thirds of Alzheimer's sufferers are women, and African Americans are twice as likely to develop it.

Genetics, diet and exercise habits, sleep patterns and a history of head trauma are all thought to play a strong role in the onset and course of Alzheimer's disease. But so, too, are the 100 trillion or so microorganisms that make up the gut microbiome. Known to influence everything from basic digestive processes to mood and emotional health, the distribution of bacteria within the colon has recently been found to be a significant factor in a range of neurodegenerative diseases, including other forms of dementia. What explains the link between microbiome health and these age-related diseases? Let's take a closer look at the connection.

From Colon to Cognition

Dementia refers to a handful of cognitive disorders that involve impairments in memory, thinking and reasoning ability. It's an umbrella term, but "almost all forms of dementia share a common denominator: brain inflammation," says William Li, MD, author of *Eat to Beat Disease: The New Science of How Your Body Can Heal Itself.* Alzheimer's—characterized by a buildup of protein fragments called beta-amyloid plaques and tangles of tau proteins inside the brain that disrupt neuronal function—is the most common and widely studied cause of dementia, accounting for up to 70 percent of all cases.

"Recent human studies have revealed distinct differences in the intestinal microbiomes of healthy individuals and those with Alzheimer's disease," says Lawrence Hoberman, MD, a gastroenterologist in San Antonio. "Individuals with Alzheimer's have a lower number and less diverse species of bacteria in their gut." This microbial imbalance is thought to trigger the immune system, causing an inflammatory response that breaks down the intestinal lining (leading to a condition known as "leaky gut"). "This releases inflammatory proteins that travel to the brain, resulting in neurologic inflammation and the production of amyloid and tau proteins," adds Hoberman.

Typically, the blood-brain barrier serves as an extremely choosy checkpoint, keeping unwanted substances that escape through a leaky gut from entering the brain, says clinical health sciences researcher Bart Wolbers. However, the blood-brain barrier can itself become increasingly permeable under certain circumstances: Age, stress and disease can cause it to let down its guard, allowing pathogens like inflammation-promoting bacteria to sneak into the brain.

"Gut microbiota can also influence brain function via the vagus nerve, the longest cranial nerve in the body, which runs from the brain to the esophagus, stomach and intestines," says Li. "Healthy and unhealthy gut bacteria can stimulate the vagus nerve in different ways, causing it to trigger the release of different neurochemicals involved in stress regulation, cognitive function, basic bodily functions like breathing and heart rate, and inflammation."

Generally speaking, the vagus nerve plays an important role in calming the body's stress response by decreasing inflammation and triggering the production of chemicals that cause the intestinal walls to tighten up (thereby improving leaky gut), Li adds. But when there's psychological, environmental or physical stress (think: anxiety, pollution or injury) the vagus nerve's functioning is dampened.

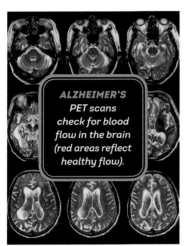

ALZHEIMER'S PET scans check for blood flow in the brain (red areas reflect healthy flow).

Healthy Habits

While improving the balance of beneficial bacteria through diet can't eliminate the risk of dementia, it may help reduce your chances —while boosting overall health. Lifestyle changes like exercise can improve blood flow to the brain and improve memory. And managing chronic conditions like high cholesterol, high blood pressure or diabetes—also plays a significant role in reducing dementia risk.

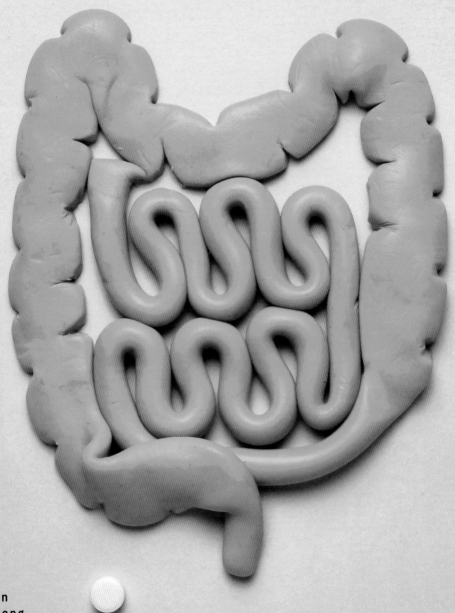

Bugs in
the wrong
spot can be
problematic.

THE ALPHABET SOUP OF

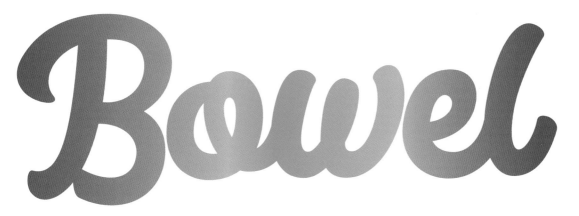

Bowel

PROBLEMS

CONFUSED BY ALL THE ACRONYMS THAT SURROUND GASTROINTESTINAL HEALTH? HERE'S HOW TO MAKE SENSE OUT OF SOME OF THE MOST COMMON DIAGNOSES.

By now, you know that what happens in the gut can potentially affect your entire body—but sometimes, what's bothering you is actually what's happening *in* the gut. Besides constipation, diarrhea, nausea and stomach pain, there's an alphabet soup of gastrointestinal tract disorders—IBD, IBS, SIBO and SIFO—that are super-common and potentially very distressing.

Give Me an I!

IBD, or inflammatory bowel disease, is an umbrella term that refers to chronic inflammation in the gastrointestinal tract. The two most common types of IBD are Crohn's disease and ulcerative colitis (UC). They're considered autoimmune disorders, although scientists are still exploring the causes and how genetics and environment may factor in. One thing is certain: An inflamed intestine is not a happy intestine. It doesn't absorb nutrients or water well, and an ulcerated lining may bleed, leading to symptoms like diarrhea, as well as blood and mucus in the stool. Both are potentially life-threatening, due to complications such as anemia and colon cancer. Blood and stool tests, as well as other screening methods, are used to help diagnose IBD.

In UC, the entire inner lining of the colon is inflamed, whereas Crohn's presents in patches of tissue. Crohn's also invades more layers of

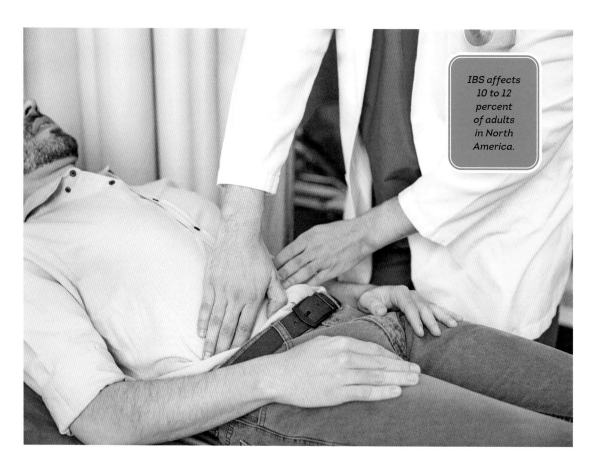

IBS affects 10 to 12 percent of adults in North America.

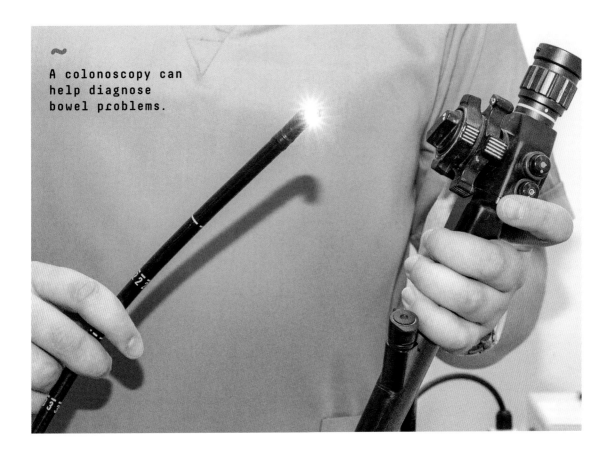

A colonoscopy can help diagnose bowel problems.

the intestinal tract and can occur at any point along the GI tract, from the mouth to the anus; it's most common in the small intestine.

As autoimmune diseases, they may also cause pain and inflammation outside the gut, such as in the joints or skin, but that is more common with Crohn's. Both conditions have "flare-ups" where symptoms get worse, then ease up. There's no cure, but both can be managed via medications, diet and, if necessary, surgery.

And Another I...

IBS, or irritable bowel syndrome, is a functional gastrointestinal disorder, or a miscommunication between the brain and gut, rather than a problem that's due to the structure of the GI tract. That's what can make it such a frustrating condition. IBS has symptoms that mimic IBD—diarrhea, constipation or a combo of both. While IBS certainly impacts quality of life, it does not result in inflammation in the GI tract. Abdominal pain or bloating that is associated with changes in stool is one key way doctors diagnose the condition. With IBS, blood tests and imaging will come back normal.

"I believe that we have not reached a level of sophistication within science to truly understand this condition," says Mel Schottenstein, NMD, chief medical officer for Crohn's Colitis Lifestyle. "The symptoms are very real, and dietary changes, probiotics and other therapies do eliminate them."

Or a C?

Like IBD, celiac disease is an autoimmune condition,but one with a known cause. About 30 to 40 percent of people carry the gene for celiac, and in about 1 percent, eating gluten—the protein found in grains such as wheat, barley and rye—destroys the intestinal villi. This results in gut damage and malnutrition, as the villi can no longer do their job absorbing nutrients as food passes through.

Celiac can be hard to pin down, as there are hundreds of possible symptoms, according to Beyond Celiac, which reports that 83 percent of patients with celiac are either misdiagnosed or not diagnosed at all. "Physicians don't turn to celiac first; they just aren't trained that way," says Marilyn G. Geller, CEO of the nonprofit Celiac Disease Foundation.

Say the word "celiac" to most people, and "they usually think of gastrointestinal symptoms: vomiting, diarrhea, constipation," says Geller. But other problems can include neuropathy, anxiety, depression, fatigue, migraines or painful canker sores. "Two biggies are unexplained anemia and early-onset osteoporosis, especially in men, who typically aren't as susceptible to osteoporosis," adds Geller. Blood tests, such as the tTG-IgA, EmA and total serum IgA, as well as endoscopies and biopsies, help doctors nail down a diagnosis.

But there is good news: Following a strict gluten-free diet can help manage the disease. It sounds simple, until you realize gluten lurks not only in breads but also in some salad dressings, soups, food coloring and more. And because going gluten-free is a food trend embraced by a wide spectrum of Americans, it can be nearly impossible to convince others (say, restaurant servers) that gluten is a genuine medical concern. "If a salad has a crouton on it, and you send it back to get a new salad and all they do is take off the crouton, that crouton dust is enough to make someone with celiac very ill," says Geller. Still, avoiding gluten can heal the gut. "It may take months or even years," stresses Geller. "But it is possible."

Try an S?

SIBO/SIFO are acronyms for small intestine bacterial (or fungal) overgrowth. Both the large and small intestine have a population of microorganisms such as streptococci, aerobic lactobacilli and fungi (there is far less in the small intestine). In SIBO, there's an overgrowth of bacteria in the small intestine, either of types that normally shouldn't be there or of types that belong, but have gotten too populous. In SIFO, there's a similar overgrowth of fungi.

SIBO/SIFO can cause symptoms such as gas, bloating, nutritional deficiencies, osteoporosis and chronic diarrhea. You may have heard more about these issues recently, but they've been around for awhile; they just weren't diagnosed as often. With so much research focusing on the gut, physicians are more aware of SIBO and SIFO, which can be diagnosed via a breath test. SIBO frequently overlaps with conditions such as Crohn's and celiac. And according to the American College of Internists, approximately 30 to 80 percent of IBS patients also have SIBO.

Both are treated in a variety of ways, including with antibiotics or antifungals, probiotics (though that is controversial), antimicrobials, and medications that make the small bowel contract more. Patients may also be steered toward a low-FODMAPs diet (see page 96).

The Last Word

If you have symptoms or a diagnosed gut disorder, seek out a gastroenterologist who handles a high volume of patients with your condition. Look for someone who works with subspecialists you may need—especially nutritionists who can guide you through various diets that can help minimize issues and heal your gut.

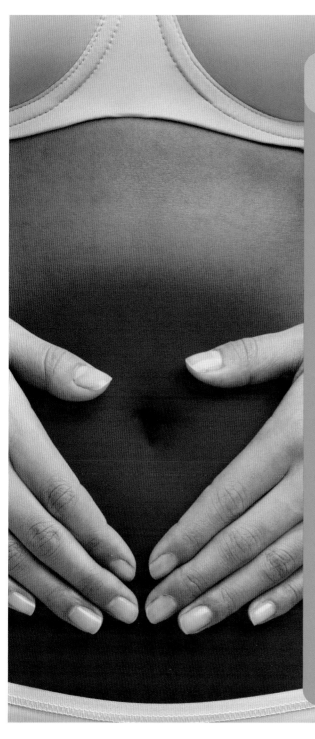

The Gut-Stress Connection

Bloating, urgent diarrhea, pain, fatigue, noxious gas, an inability to poop for days: Bowel disorders can seriously impact your lifestyle and cause a huge amount of stress, which in turn makes symptoms worse. Psychological stress can significantly impair the intestines' ability to move food along, secrete enzymes and hormones, and absorb nutrients. It can also activate the gut immune system and alter the microbiome, according to the Mayo Clinic. Stress-management techniques, such as visualization, hypnosis and therapy, can in some cases turn down the volume on symptoms— especially when it comes to IBS. But for other conditions, they can at least help reduce the anxiety and depression that frequently accompany chronic GI issues.

"Psychological interventions are well-established, effective treatments for IBS, and cognitive behavior therapy [CBT] in particular has been rigorously tested in clinical trials and consistently demonstrates significant and long-lasting symptom improvement," according to a 2017 study published in Psychology Research and Behavior Management. *More recent research (published in the journal* Gut*) even found that working with a web-based or telephone-based CBT therapist improved quality of life for IBS sufferers, which could open up access to many more patients.*

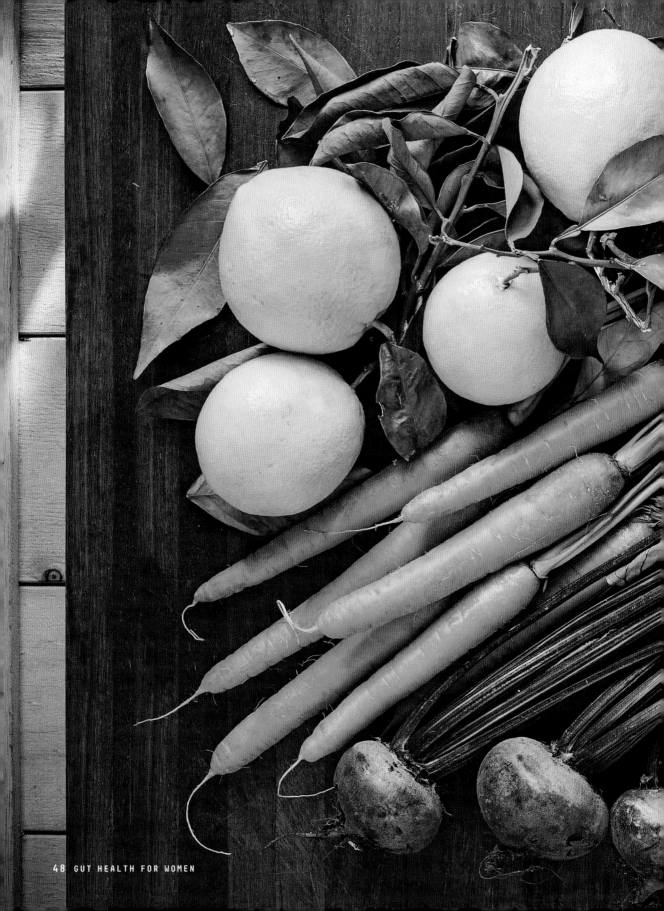

2

How to
Feed
Your Bugs

*HATS OFF TO HIPPOCRATES, WHO FAMOUSLY SAID,
"LET FOOD BE THY MEDICINE AND MEDICINE BE THY FOOD" — AND
HE WAS RIGHT. THE CURE FOR MANY HEALTH ISSUES,
INCLUDING ECZEMA, HEART DISEASE, DIABETES AND DEPRESSION,
REALLY DOES START WITH YOUR DIET.*

THE TRUTH ABOUT
Probiotics

YOU'VE PROBABLY HEARD A LOT ABOUT THESE "GOOD" BACTERIA. NOW LEARN THE FACTS.

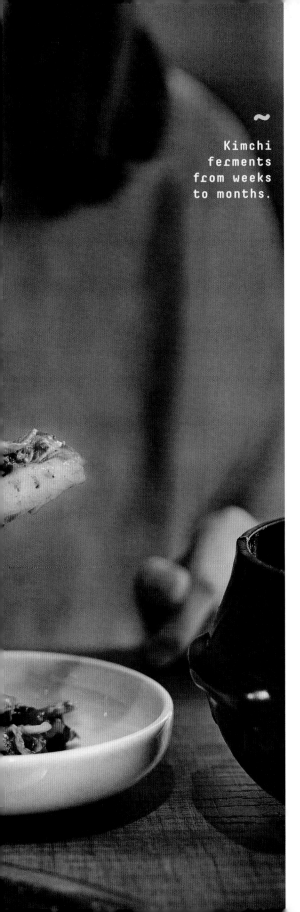

Kimchi
ferments
from weeks
to months.

here is no such thing as a magic pill, but many people seem convinced that probiotics come pretty close. Now marketed for everything from gastrointestinal distress to mental health to skin problems, probiotics not only take up major real estate in the supplement aisle, they've also leaped from yogurt and kombucha to flavored waters, protein powders, granola and more.

"In the past 15 to 20 years, people have really been going back to understanding what is in food nutritionally and how it impacts our health," says nutritional microbiologist David Sela, PhD, professor of food science at the University of Massachusetts Amherst. "Beneficial microbes used to ferment foods are considered by some to be probiotic. We are clever enough to capture them and put them into supplements to our advantage, and companies do a great job of marketing them."

But for all the hype, there's still so much we don't know about how probiotics work, which ones are best for what conditions and whether taking a supplement will do anything for you. So before you buy any pill or food with added probiotics, read on to learn what experts—and the growing body of research—have to say.

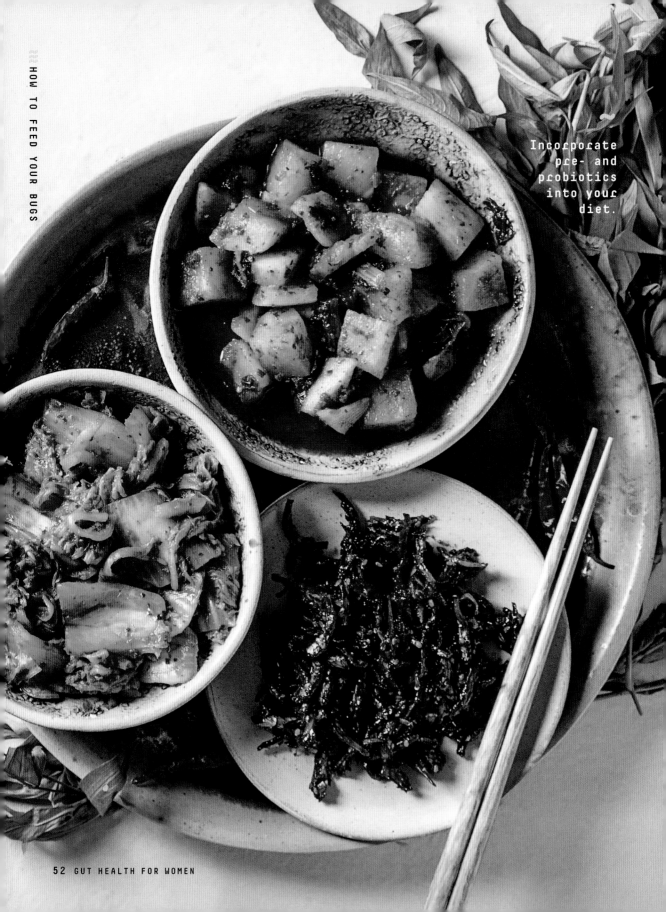

Incorporate
pre- and
probiotics
into your
diet.

Hard-Working Bugs

Probiotics are generally described as "good" bacteria, and that's a fairly accurate definition. "The word 'probiotic' comes from Greek—'pro' meaning 'for' and 'bios' meaning 'life,'" explains functional-medicine doctor Vincent Pedre, MD, author of *Happy Gut: The Cleansing Program to Help You Lose Weight, Gain Energy and Eliminate Pain.* "The idea is that they are beneficial to use and believed to have a positive effect on our health in some way."

Probiotics are found naturally in the gut as well as in certain foods, and the probiotics in supplements are similar to those in your gut. These live, active microbes help digest food, destroy disease-causing microorganisms and produce vitamins. They also promote a healthy balance of "good" and "bad" bacteria in the colon. Your goal isn't to wipe out the bad bacteria; you just don't want too many of them. "The gut is like a rain forest," Pedre explains. "Even a predator must be fulfilling some role and serving to keep balance within the ecosystem. So in any healthy gut, there will be a certain percentage of unfavorable, or pathogenic, bacteria."

Many experts believe this improved gut-bacteria balance may help improve your health. However, if your GI system is already working well, you may not experience any changes if you add probiotic supplements to your routine (i.e., more isn't better).

The Possible Pros

When scientists perform meta-analyses on research, they generally find a benefit from taking probiotics, says Emeran Mayer, MD, PhD, author of *The Mind-Gut Connection* and a professor of medicine and psychiatry in UCLA's division of digestive diseases. "Health or wellness benefits are almost impossible to study in traditional clinical trials," he adds. "From my experience in my clinic, you can see a benefit in about 10 to 15 percent of patients who are taking them. Probiotics have a small benefit on a wide variety of diseases in the GI tract, but they're not a magic pill."

But there is no one probiotic that works for everyone or everything. "There is evidence for specific probiotics to have a specific beneficial effect in specific populations of people against specific outcomes," says Sela. "Things have to line up just right." With that in mind, probiotics may have benefits for the following:

There are up to

1,000

different species of bacteria living in the gastrointestinal tract.

DIARRHEA

Probiotics appear to help with both infectious and antibiotic-associated diarrhea, perhaps the best-known benefit from research so far. In a Cochrane review of 63 studies, researchers found that taking probiotics (in food or supplements) shortened the duration of acute infectious diarrhea by about a day, and lessened the risk of the symptoms lasting four or more days by 59 percent. A more recent review of 36 studies on antibiotic-associated diarrhea in children found that probiotics—especially 5 to 40 billion colony forming units (CFU) of Lactobacillus rhamnosus or Saccharomyces

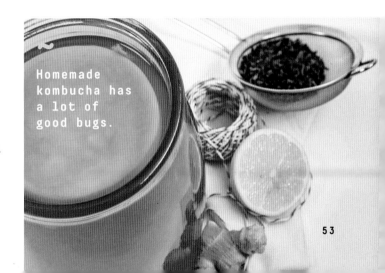

Homemade kombucha has a lot of good bugs.

boulardii per day—can prevent one case of diarrhea for every nine children treated.

CONSTIPATION

If your problem is not that you go too much but that you can't go, probiotics may help, too. In a meta-analysis of 14 randomized controlled studies published in the *American Journal of Clinical Nutrition*, probiotics reduced gut transit time by almost 12.5 hours, increased stool frequency by 1.3 times per week and softened stools. Probiotics containing Bifidobacterium appeared to be most effective. However, the study authors add that more research is necessary, as the papers in the analysis varied widely in their designs and results.

PRO TIP
Change up your "bug" supplement every few months.

OTHER GASTROINTESTINAL ISSUES

Whether you have medically diagnosed irritable bowel syndrome (IBS) or simply experience symptoms such as abdominal pain, bloating, gas and distension, there's mixed evidence that probiotics may help. For example, while a 2016 review by the British Dietetic Association found probiotics improved at least one symptom in 83 percent of the 35 trials analyzed, the authors concluded it is too premature to make specific recommendations. However, the authors of a 2018 paper in *Foods* concluded that multistrain probiotics at a concentration of 10 billion CFU for a day or less appear to offer the "best chance of improving abdominal pain, global symptoms and...quality of life in IBS sufferers."

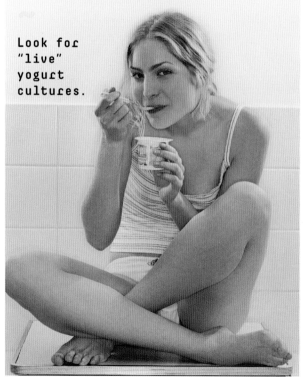

Look for "live" yogurt cultures.

ANTIBIOTICS SIDE EFFECTS

A highly publicized yet small study printed in the journal *Cell* in 2018 reported that taking probiotics to counter the effects of antibiotics actually *delayed* gut recovery to the pre-antibiotic state by more than five months. Still, many probiotic advocates endorse taking supplements after a course of antibiotics or at the same time. "I recommend supplements, like Saccharomyces boulardii, during and after antibiotic therapy in order to restore the gut flora," says Pedre. "In my clinical experience, I have found this works quite nicely in helping patients get through antibiotic therapy and recover their gut microbiome afterward. Probiotic foods serve a benefit here post-antibiotic therapy, but are not enough to restore the gut environment."

LEAKY GUT SYNDROME

The gut barrier, which is the lining of the intestines, controls what is absorbed into the bloodstream. "If the barrier is too permeable,

PROBIOTICS SUPPLEMENT CHECKLIST

Although most experts recommend consuming probiotics from foods first, supplements may have a place. "If a person is really sick in terms of having imbalanced gut flora, they will need a probiotic supplement," says functional-medicine doctor Vincent Pedre, MD. "Or if they have a lot of yeast overgrowth, they may not be able to tolerate fermented foods, which may cause uncomfortable GI symptoms." If you choose to go the supplement route, here's what to look for—and what to avoid.

1 Pick the Right Strain

Talk to your doctor, who can help you identify which strains—and dose (in CFU)—appear to be most beneficial for the specific condition you wish to address. Then choose a supplement that contains that strain (possibly in combination with others). The CFU will likely be a number in the billions, but higher isn't necessarily better, so follow your doctor's advice. (People with "serious underlying medical problems" may want to avoid probiotics, according to the National Institutes of Health.)

2 Be Sure You Can Stomach It

"A lot of bacteria can die in the stomach," Pedre says. "You want to take a probiotic in an acid-stable capsule so it can resist stomach acid and get into the small bowel and large intestine where it's needed." Check the label (or call the company) for the words "acid-resistant."

4 Check the Expiration Date

"As soon as probiotics are encapsulated, they start to degrade," Pedre says. The CFUs on the label indicate how many survive until the expiration date. (Not that you should wait that long to take them.)

3 Decide if You Need to Chill

Refrigerated probiotics aren't necessarily better than shelf-stable ones, especially if you travel often. However, if you choose the latter, be sure they come in blister packs. "This means they're packaged in a nitrogen environment [with minimal oxygen inside] to keep the probiotics viable until you break open the blister," Pedre explains.

5 Seal It In

Look for a seal from a third-party verification program—such as NSF International or USP—to guarantee that the product contains what the label says it does, in those amounts, and also contains no contaminants.

Healthy lifestyle habits trump pills.

toxins can enter the body and lead to all sorts of inflammatory reactions," Pedre says. "An influx of endotoxins is associated with obesity, weight gain, pre-diabetes and metabolic syndrome. In fact, many of the metabolic disorders we thought were hormone-based may actually be controlled by bacteria in the gut." Taking probiotics may help preserve the integrity of the GI tract and prevent leaky gut syndrome.

OTHER CONDITIONS

As for other benefits of probiotics, "it's an evolving science, and there is a lot we're still learning," Pedre says. This includes how probiotics affect the immune system, mental health and diabetes, as well as how they might improve the gut flora of someone who has an unbalanced microbiome and the role of different gut bacteria in different diseases.

Food for Thought

Despite all of these potential benefits, hold off before you rush to buy a bottle of probiotic supplements, as most experts recommend food first. And to really ensure a healthy gut, you also need to consume prebiotics, a type of fiber that probiotics eat, says Sela.

"My recommendation is to increase the amount of naturally fermented foods in your diet and to eat different types of foods," says Mayer. This includes kombucha (with minimal added sugars), kimchi, kefir and some yogurts, and sauerkraut. "A variety of probiotic strains and species from different sources seems to be a more prudent approach, although there is no hard science on this," adds Mayer, who recommends downing fermented foods as part of a regular, mainly plant-based, health-promoting diet.

Postbiotics: A New Frontier

Postbiotics are "the byproducts produced when probiotics ferment prebiotics in the gut," says dietitian Kara Landau. These byproducts include peptides, enzymes and short-chain fatty acids (SCFAs), such as butyrate. "It's really the postbiotics—not the probiotics—that ultimately lead to gut health benefits," Landau adds. For example, eating a diet rich in fiber increases the production of butyrate, which in turn may affect inflammation in the gut and brain. There's also evidence that SCFAs play a role in insulin sensitivity, glucose metabolism and immunity, and also may have anti-tumor effects, among other benefits.

At this point, though, the research on postbiotic health benefits is very early, and there's no consensus on the definition of "postbiotics." Researchers need that so the field can be regulated and scientists can properly link postbiotics to their specific health benefits.

You can find them in food: "You can eat butyrate, but it tastes like vomit," says Iowa State researcher Thomas Mansell, PhD. So the best way to get postbiotics in your diet is to eat foods that are already rich in prebiotics.

You can find them in supplements: There are products containing postbiotics on the market, but hold off on trying any of them. "I like the idea because it could allow you to more reliably deliver the molecules that are doing good," Mansell says. "But that's very reductionist." It's the same as trying to isolate a specific micronutrient, like a vitamin in a fruit: Taking that vitamin in isolation often doesn't lead to the same health benefit that consuming the whole food does.

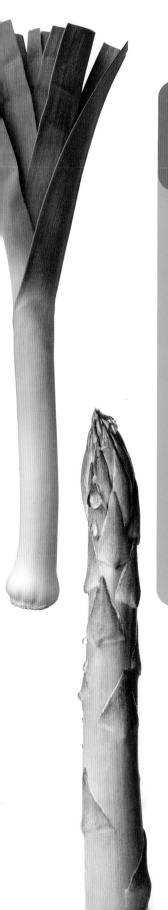

The Microbiome Set Point: Back to Square One?

Some scientists have begun to discuss a gut microbiome "set point." While there is no firm definition of this colloquial term, "my interpretation of 'set point' is the way in which our gut microbiome is both resilient—typically returning to its normal state following a disturbance—and also individually specific," says Katerina Johnson, PhD, a research associate at the University of Oxford. (Although long-term studies are necessary, this sort of homeostasis appears to be established within the first two years of life.)

For example, research suggests that even if you take antibiotics, have gastroenteritis from food poisoning, or temporarily change your diet and then return to a normal way of eating, "our gut microbiome can normally recover from these disturbances after awhile to resemble its composition before the disturbance," Johnson explains.

That's usually a good thing—but not always. Does this mean that taking probiotics in an effort to shift your microbiome composition is all for naught? Evidence is still lacking, Johnson says. "However, just because a probiotic may not be able to colonize the gut, it does not necessarily mean it cannot affect the body's physiology as it passes through," she adds.

And each person's microbiome may respond differently to dietary changes. Still, changing how you eat can shift your gut microbiome composition in the long term (as can exercise and managing stress). "Diet seems to be the most direct link to naturally bring about changes to the gut," says Johnson. Just stick with it. "If you increase the fiber you're eating and then return to your normal diet, the composition of your gut microbiome would be expected to return to its previous state."

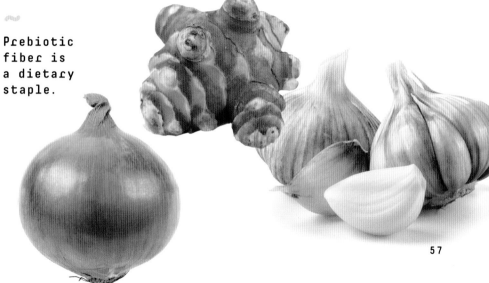

Prebiotic fiber is a dietary staple.

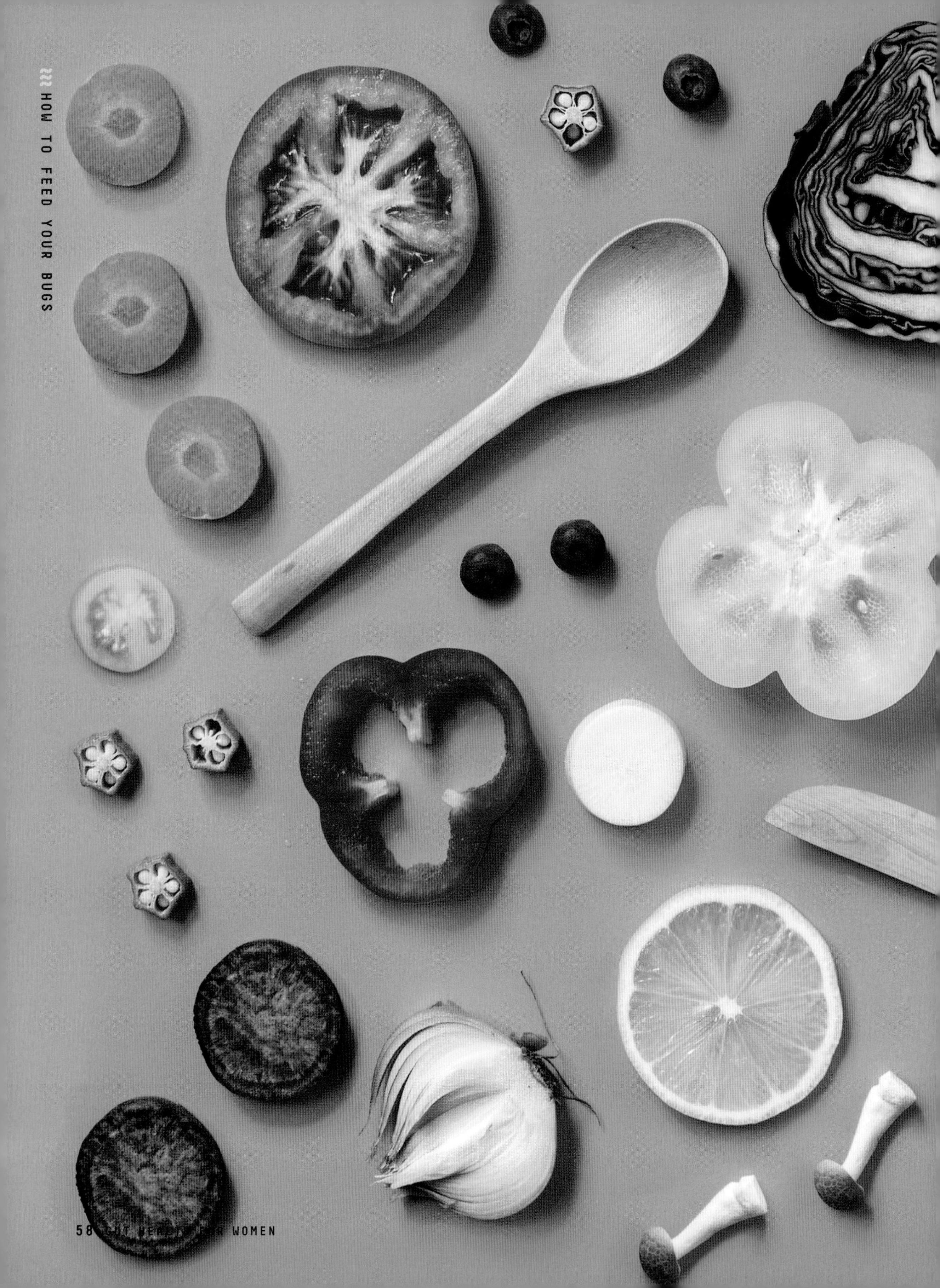

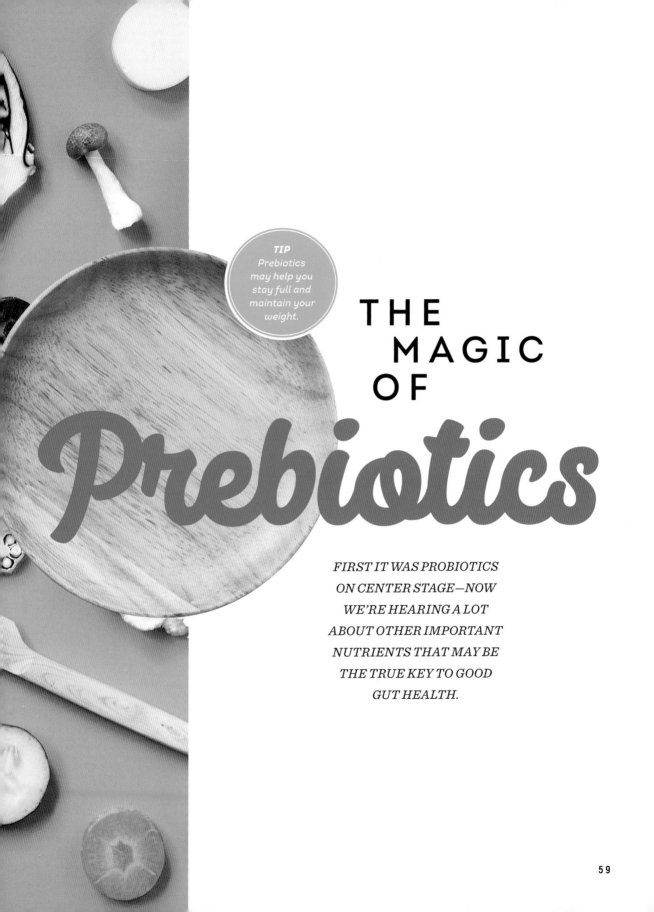

TIP
Prebiotics may help you stay full and maintain your weight.

THE MAGIC OF *Prebiotics*

FIRST IT WAS PROBIOTICS ON CENTER STAGE—NOW WE'RE HEARING A LOT ABOUT OTHER IMPORTANT NUTRIENTS THAT MAY BE THE TRUE KEY TO GOOD GUT HEALTH.

Pre-, pro-, postbiotics: There are a lot of prefixes to keep track of these days when it comes to eating for healthy digestion, but the differences are important. Probiotics are the living microorganisms—especially the 1,000 species of bacteria—that reside in the GI tract. Over the past decade, scientists have been discovering how these little guys boost the immune system, help maintain healthy skin, decrease depression and anxiety, and even alter how you react to medications. But like any living thing, these organisms need to eat, and that's where prebiotics come in.

According to one definition published in the journal *Nutrients*, a prebiotic is an ingredient that makes it to the colon without being digested; is fermented by the intestinal microbes; and stimulates the bacteria to promote health and well-being (they produce postbiotics, which the body uses for various functions).

"Prebiotics are essentially just dietary fiber, although some colleagues maintain the opinion that there are inherent differences—meaning, prebiotics are fermented by specific microbes, while fibers are not," says Jens Walter, PhD, an associate professor and a specialist in nutrition, microbes and gastrointestinal health at the University of Alberta in Canada. "There is a saying that all prebiotics are fibers, but not all fibers are prebiotics. For me, the value of prebiotics is that they provide growth substrates to gut microbiota, and by doing so, support fermentation in the gut, which is associated with beneficial metabolic outcomes."

But different types of dietary fiber do work in different ways. Walter notes, "Viscous fibers such as beta-glucan lower cholesterol, while other fibers do so on a lesser scale." Research published in the journal *Nature*

Diet changes show up in the gut quickly.

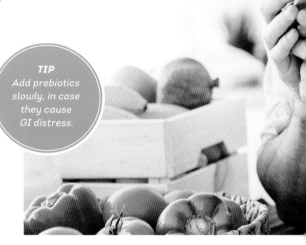

TIP
Add prebiotics slowly, in case they cause GI distress.

found that a type of fiber called inulin supported a surprisingly broad boost in the volume and diversity of gut microbes.

And a study published in the *Journal of Animal Science and Biotechnology* emphasizes that fermentability of fiber affects how gut microbes respond. It also argues that while the colon has been considered the most important place for prebiotics to work their magic, "it is slowly being recognized that while there are fewer microbial numbers and activity in the stomach and small intestine, the activity occurring here is also likely to be relevant."

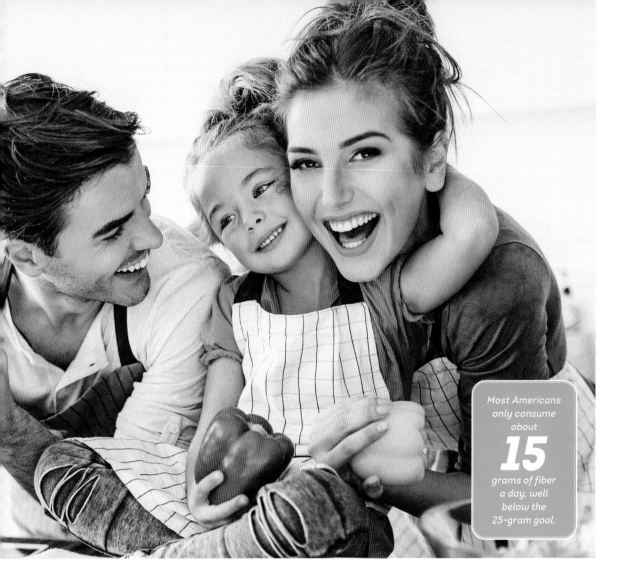

Most Americans only consume about **15** grams of fiber a day, well below the 25-gram goal.

Going to the Source

Prebiotics are found naturally in whole grains and vegetables, and can also be purchased in supplement form. The less refined the source, the better, says Jenna Hollenstein, RDN, a New York City–based nutrition therapist and author of the book *Eat to Love*. "Look for bananas, dark leafy greens, artichokes, Jerusalem artichokes, garlic and onions," she says. The latter two can cause gas, bloating or discomfort for some people, so if you're sensitive, there are plenty of other options for prebiotics, including apples, jicama, watermelon and oats. The interesting thing, Hollenstein says, is that consuming enough prebiotics may help the gut rebalance to the point that foods that used to trigger sensitivities are better tolerated.

"The gut is complex, personalized and constantly changing, and like many parts of our experience, is affected by both physical and mental factors," says Hollenstein. To make a difference, prebiotics need to be a regular part of the diet, not a one-time, "eat a bowl and you're set" situation.

Despite their significance, there is currently no RDA for prebiotics, but the U.S. Dietary

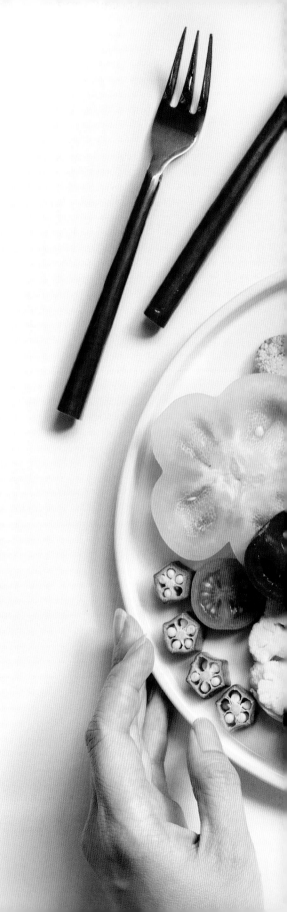

Guidelines do recommend eating 25 grams of fiber a day for women and 38 grams for men. Most Americans only down half that amount.

Popular keto or gluten-free diets may also be insufficient in prebiotics. "Some of these diets are very heavy on protein and fat, and don't necessarily promote consuming whole grains, fruits or vegetables," says Bruce Y. Lee, MD, a professor of health policy and management at City University of New York. Even a healthy-seeming juice cleanse may present challenges. "The science of making processed foods is moving faster than the science of knowing what we are doing," says Lee. "For hundreds and thousands of years, human bodies were used to eating fruits and vegetables. Is liquid the same as eating it whole? There is evidence it's not the same, even if it's green stuff, even if it's all natural. Eating a prebiotic as a powder is different from eating a plant. Try to minimize the processing of the food you're eating."

Besides depriving your beneficial bacteria of their favorite food, falling short on prebiotics in the gut can worsen certain GI conditions, too. "I have known of people who are on these very restrictive diets specifically because of GI issues, like IBS, bloating or constipation," says Hollenstein. "Ironically, they may be moving further away from prebiotics, therefore exacerbating their condition, as their colonies of gut bacteria will be really diminished."

The Takeaway

As with gut research in general, many studies on prebiotics were conducted on animals, not humans, so the jury is out on many details. While there are differences of opinion, the scientists we spoke to all agree in several areas: You should eat a variety of prebiotics from a variety of food groups and in their natural state whenever possible.

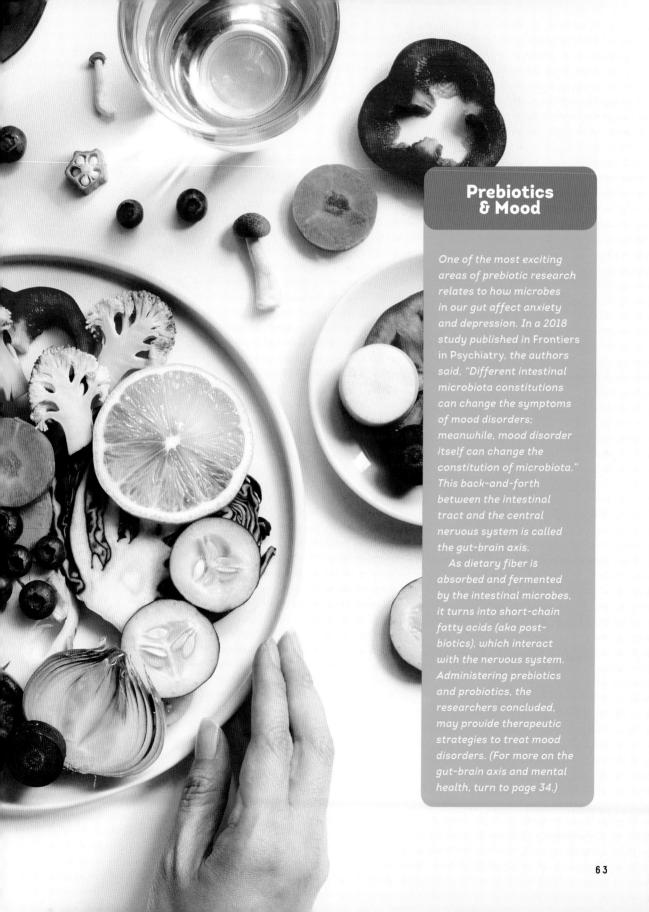

Prebiotics & Mood

One of the most exciting areas of prebiotic research relates to how microbes in our gut affect anxiety and depression. In a 2018 study published in Frontiers in Psychiatry, *the authors said, "Different intestinal microbiota constitutions can change the symptoms of mood disorders; meanwhile, mood disorder itself can change the constitution of microbiota."* This back-and-forth between the intestinal tract and the central nervous system is called the gut-brain axis.

As dietary fiber is absorbed and fermented by the intestinal microbes, it turns into short-chain fatty acids (aka post-biotics), which interact with the nervous system. Administering prebiotics and probiotics, the researchers concluded, may provide therapeutic strategies to treat mood disorders. (For more on the gut-brain axis and mental health, turn to page 34.)

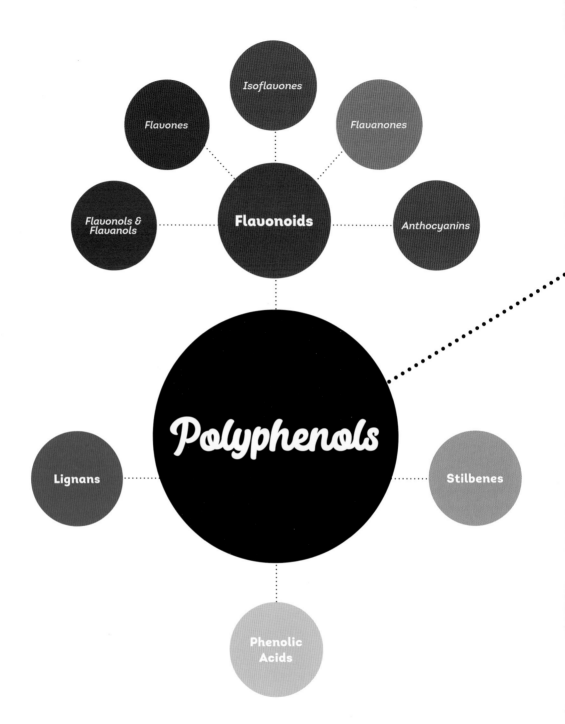

THESE PLANT CHEMICALS MAY HAVE THE POWER TO INCREASE GOOD
GUT BACTERIA, FIGHT FREE RADICALS AND BOOST YOUR HEALTH.

Phenoms of the Plant World

THE FAMILY TREE Polyphenols are one of the most numerous and widely distributed natural compounds in the plant kingdom. Scientists have identified more than 8,000 polyphenols, and classify them based on their phenolic groups and structural elements. Even these can be confusing, as the classes also have subclasses (see diagram, opposite).

What do berries, onions, tea, chocolate, coffee and beer all have in common? Yes, all are delicious, but they're also all sources of polyphenols, phytochemicals—"phyto" means derived from plants—that researchers are studying for their ability to improve the gut microbiota and potentially spur further-reaching health perks, too. "Polyphenols are compounds that interact with different processes in our bodies when we metabolize our food," says Hannah Cory, RD, a PhD candidate in the nutrition department at the Harvard T.H. Chan School of Public Health. "Research shows they may have a lot of potential impacts on disease for humans."

You may have heard the terms flavonoids, isoflavones and anthocyanins, which are all polyphenols with their own specific functions and benefits. Although researchers continue to learn more about these ubiquitous compounds, one thing we do know is that they are antioxidants. Think of them as scavengers searching for free radicals, which are unstable, highly active atoms that cause damage, inflammation and illness in the body. Polyphenols find and then negate free radicals, which prevents them from doing any harm. "Cardiovascular disease, metabolic syndrome, cognitive decline, cancers—a lot of these health issues are linked with inflammation, so if we can address that, it's a big deal," says nutritional microbiologist David Sela, PhD, professor of food science at the University of Massachusetts Amherst.

POLY-POWERFUL

If you're eating a plant-based diet, you're likely consuming a good number of polyphenols already, since they're found in a variety of fruits, vegetables, nuts and legumes. If not, read on to find out why you should be adding them to your menu ASAP.

1 Improved Gut Function

In a study published in *The Journal of Nutritional Biochemistry*, scientists fed mice either a regular diet or one high in fat. Half of each group also consumed green tea extract, which is high in catechins, a type of anti-inflammatory polyphenol. In both diet groups, the green tea appeared to support a healthier gut microbiome, leading to stronger, less "leaky" guts. However, this effect was stronger for those fed the high-fat, green tea–fortified diet. The scientists in part credit the polyphenols.

They not only seem to stimulate the growth of good bacteria; polyphenols also appear to inhibit the growth of bad bacteria, according to a review published in *The Journal of Nutritional Biochemistry.* "There seems to be a two-way street between gut health and polyphenols," Cory says. "A lot of processing of nutrients goes on in the large intestine, and whether or not you absorb polyphenols might depend on your gut bacteria. On the flip side, there is research showing they may help boost microbiome health. So it might be a feedback loop." (Healthier bacteria are better able to absorb polyphenols.)

2 Brain Benefits

These positive changes in the gut may also have neuroprotective perks. We now know that the gut and brain have a bidirectional relationship (see page 34). Some researchers believe that since polyphenols support healthy gut microbiota, they may also support a healthy brain—and even prevent neurodegeneration and diseases such as Parkinson's and Alzheimer's. "One idea is that polyphenols might prevent neurotoxicity," Cory explains. This happens when natural or man-made toxic substances alter normal nervous system activity—including that of the brain.

3 Cardiovascular Health

In addition to fighting inflammation, foods rich in flavonoids may help lower blood pressure, reduce platelet activity and decrease "bad" LDL cholesterol. Polyphenols also appear to increase the amount of nitric oxide in the body, which helps regulate the cardiovascular, immune and nervous systems, Cory says. Low levels of nitric oxide are associated with damage that occurs in the lining of the blood vessels, which is a hallmark of cardiovascular diseases. "It also helps signal blood vessels to dilate, so some polyphenols may help with blood flow and pressure," Cory adds.

4 Cancer Prevention

Research shows that free-radical damage to cells and DNA may play a role in the development of cancer. Polyphenols found in soy, called isoflavones, are well-known for their anti-cancer properties. But the list of potential cancer-fighting polyphenols also includes flavonoids, anthocyanins, catechins, flavonols, flavones, flavanones and isoflavones, all of which appear to neutralize free radicals. "Polyphenols can act like a cleanup crew," Cory says. "They're scavenging and picking up things that might be bad in the body."

5 Enhanced Longevity

Italian researchers followed 807 adults for 12 years and measured their polyphenol intake by analyzing their urine. They found that those who consumed the highest levels of polyphenols also lived longer. The study authors believe this may be due to the fact that polyphenol intake is inversely associated with chronic health conditions such as cardiovascular disease, cancer and neurodegenerative diseases.

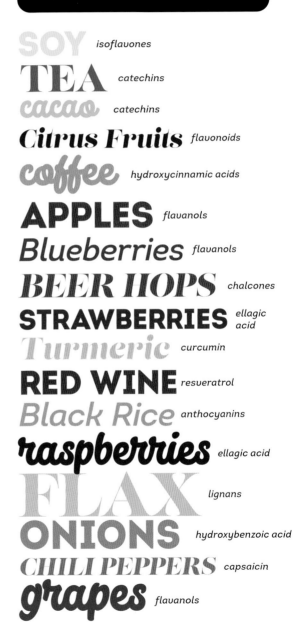

What's in a Name?
Many plant foods have polyphenols, and most contain multiple types. While by no means comprehensive, here are some of the polyphenols found in common foods.

SOY — *isoflavones*

TEA — *catechins*

cacao — *catechins*

Citrus Fruits — *flavonoids*

coffee — *hydroxycinnamic acids*

APPLES — *flavanols*

Blueberries — *flavanols*

BEER HOPS — *chalcones*

STRAWBERRIES — *ellagic acid*

Turmeric — *curcumin*

RED WINE — *resveratrol*

Black Rice — *anthocyanins*

raspberries — *ellagic acid*

FLAX — *lignans*

ONIONS — *hydroxybenzoic acid*

CHILI PEPPERS — *capsaicin*

grapes — *flavanols*

~

Add fruit to meals to ease digestion. Bananas, kiwi, mango, papaya and pineapple contain enzymes that break down protein, fat or carbohydrates.

Supplements You Can Stomach

BEYOND PROBIOTICS AND A HEALTHIER DIET, THERE ARE MANY PRODUCTS THAT CAN HELP YOUR DIGESTIVE TRACT RUN SMOOTHLY.

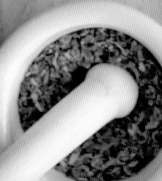

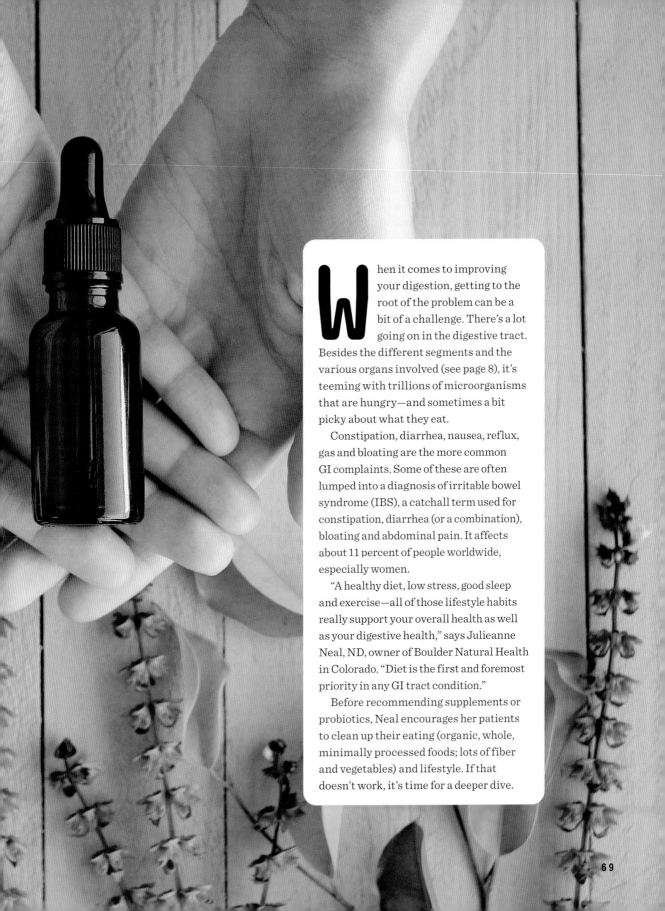

When it comes to improving your digestion, getting to the root of the problem can be a bit of a challenge. There's a lot going on in the digestive tract. Besides the different segments and the various organs involved (see page 8), it's teeming with trillions of microorganisms that are hungry—and sometimes a bit picky about what they eat.

Constipation, diarrhea, nausea, reflux, gas and bloating are the more common GI complaints. Some of these are often lumped into a diagnosis of irritable bowel syndrome (IBS), a catchall term used for constipation, diarrhea (or a combination), bloating and abdominal pain. It affects about 11 percent of people worldwide, especially women.

"A healthy diet, low stress, good sleep and exercise—all of those lifestyle habits really support your overall health as well as your digestive health," says Julieanne Neal, ND, owner of Boulder Natural Health in Colorado. "Diet is the first and foremost priority in any GI tract condition."

Before recommending supplements or probiotics, Neal encourages her patients to clean up their eating (organic, whole, minimally processed foods; lots of fiber and vegetables) and lifestyle. If that doesn't work, it's time for a deeper dive.

Consider the Pros

Probiotic supplements that contain live bacteria and yeast that support the microbiome are one way to tackle gut health. Lactobacillus acidophilus and Bifidobacteria bifidum are two strains that have been shown to help with digestive issues. Experts recommend taking a broad-spectrum probiotic—with approximately 12 to 15 different strains of bugs—and no less than 5 billion CFUs—for general digestive health. It's also good to rotate brands so you're colonizing the colon with different microbes, which builds a more robust immune system. In addition, support your gut by adding fermented products, such as yogurt or sauerkraut, to your diet (see page 50 for more on probiotics).

"Probiotics are wonderful for making a more robust and diverse microbiome, but they have to be seen in context of your diet and health history," says Amy Rothenberg, ND, co-founder of the Naturopathic Health Care clinic in Northampton, Massachusetts. It's not a one-size-fits-all approach, so it's important to identify the cause of your complaints first.

Beyond Probiotics

"People reach for probiotics and gut enzymes [to aid digestion], but sometimes they can make you feel worse," says Neal. This is especially true if you have small intestine bacterial overgrowth, or SIBO, which occurs when bugs escape their cozy home in the large intestine and encroach on the small intestine, causing gas, bloating and bowel changes. Probiotics and enzymes will only serve to feed the overgrowth of bacteria, instead of working to get rid of it. For SIBO, "you'll need something to tamper down the bacteria, and then you can work on repopulating the microbiome with good bacteria," says Neal. She likes antimicrobial remedies, such as berberine or oregano oil (these can also be used for treating diarrhea).

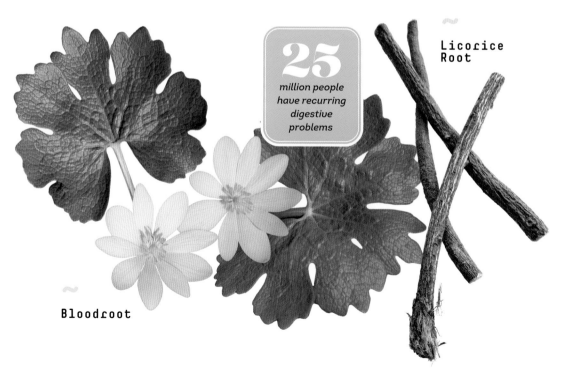

25 million people have recurring digestive problems

Licorice Root

Bloodroot

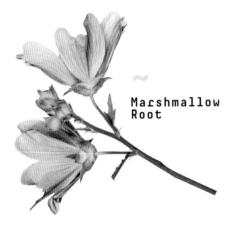

Marshmallow
Root

"But first, if you have digestive issues, speak to a medical professional about it," suggests Neal. They can rule out any organic causes. In many cases, there's not a specific reason you can point to, and that's where supplements and other treatments can help. "Natural medicine plays a role at the forefront of digestive health issues because there aren't a lot of good options or drugs in conventional health care," says Neal. "We have a huge arsenal and a variety of treatments to improve the overall health of the entire body."

Whether it's reflux, IBS or an ulcer, try these recommendations from Neal and Rothenberg. Both note that dosage is specific to each person, which is why you should consult with an expert before taking a supplement.

GI Soothers

These act like anti-inflammatories to help calm and heal the lining of the digestive tract, which can become inflamed and irritated by acid, allergens or constant constipation or diarrhea.

DEGLYCYRRHIZINATED LICORICE ROOT EXTRACT Known as DGL, this herb is what's called a demulcent or a mucoprotective agent. It helps reduce inflammation, promote a mucus barrier, and soothe the linings of the stomach, intestines and even the esophagus. A study published in *The BMJ* lauded DGL for its mucosal healing properties and found it helped neutralize or suppress gastric acid and stimulate the body's defense mechanisms

to prevent ulcers. Another study, published in the *Journal of the Australian Traditional-Medicine Society*, found that DGL was more effective than drugs that suppress acid.

MARSHMALLOW ROOT For at least 2,000 years, marshmallow root has been used in digestive healing formulas to soothe, moisten and heal intestinal mucus membranes. It's thought that the mucus produced by marshmallow root helps protect the lining of the digestive tract, decreasing the risk of some ulcers. Similarly, it also can coat the esophagus and protect it from stomach acid.

SLIPPERY ELM Derived from the bark of a tree native to the central and eastern United States and Canada, slippery elm, like DGL, is also a demulcent. Studies have shown that slippery elm bark can help to reduce the inflammation and symptoms associated with irritable bowel syndrome, and with ulcerative colitis and Crohn's disease, two types of irritable bowel disease.

Track Your Symptoms

If you're having digestive troubles, keep a food diary for two weeks. Log everything you eat (and the times) and when you notice symptoms arising. This alone might help you spot a problem, but if you're still stumped, take the log to your doctor or a nutritionist, who can help you narrow down the problem. It might be as simple as cutting back on those "sugar-free" jelly beans (which often contain sugar alcohols that can trigger gas and bloating) or opting for a product to help you digest lactose, a sugar in milk.

Bug Busters

Antibiotics can be used to tackle the overgrowth of bacteria found in SIBO, but they come with serious side effects. Natural antimicrobials, on the other hand, have been shown to inhibit bacteria, yeast/fungi and viruses, all of which reside in the gut (antibiotics only kill bacteria).

BERBERINE This alkaloid (a compound extracted from plants) is found in a variety of herbs that have been used for centuries in Chinese and Ayurvedic medicine. Berberine has antimicrobial properties and it can be just as effective as—and gentler than—antibiotics in countering bacterial overgrowth that's a staple in GI infections such as SIBO.

OREGANO OIL Thought to help protect the GI tract lining, oregano oil contains phenols, terpenes and terpenoids, all of which have strong antioxidant properties. One phenol, carvacrol, has been shown to stop the growth of different types of bacteria. In a study with people who had gut parasites, oregano oil helped kill off the bugs and eliminated symptoms in the majority of participants.

PEPPERMINT OIL Just like a cup of peppermint tea can help with indigestion, enteric-coated peppermint oil is thought to help boost overall digestive health. It has been shown to help alleviate gas and IBS symptoms such as pain and bloating by helping to relax the muscles in the colon and dull pain receptors. "Peppermint is a carminative herb," says Neal. "The volatile oil helps increase gastric emptying and peristalsis and has an antispasmodic effect on intestinal tissue." It also has antimicrobial properties and is recommended in the treatment of SIBO for its ability to inhibit bacteria growth. While not all supplements need to be enteric-coated, peppermint should be because it's a strong volatile oil, explains Neal.

Other Little Helpers

DIGESTIVE ENZYMES These chemical kick-starters found in the saliva and throughout the digestive tract help break down proteins, carbs and fats. As you age, you produce fewer digestive enzymes, so sometimes you need an extra boost. Use them if you experience indigestion, and especially if you have gas and bloating.

GINGER "Ginger is a carminative herb that helps to relieve gas," says Rothenberg. It's also an anti-inflammatory and helps relieve nausea. Try slicing ginger into wedges and making a tea with it, or grating it into food to help with nausea.

L-GLUTAMINE "This amino acid may help with a lot of different problems in the digestive system," says Rothenberg. Try it to calm the lining of the digestive tract, especially for those who suffer from chronic diarrhea or who may be undergoing chemotherapy. It serves as a building block for proteins and plays a key role in maintaining healthy cells in the gut lining.

MELATONIN While it's best known as a sleep aid, it has also been shown to help strengthen the sphincter between the esophagus and stomach, which can help with reflux. (Take it at night, or you'll feel like a zombie.)

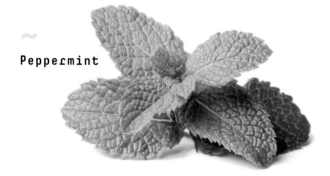
Peppermint

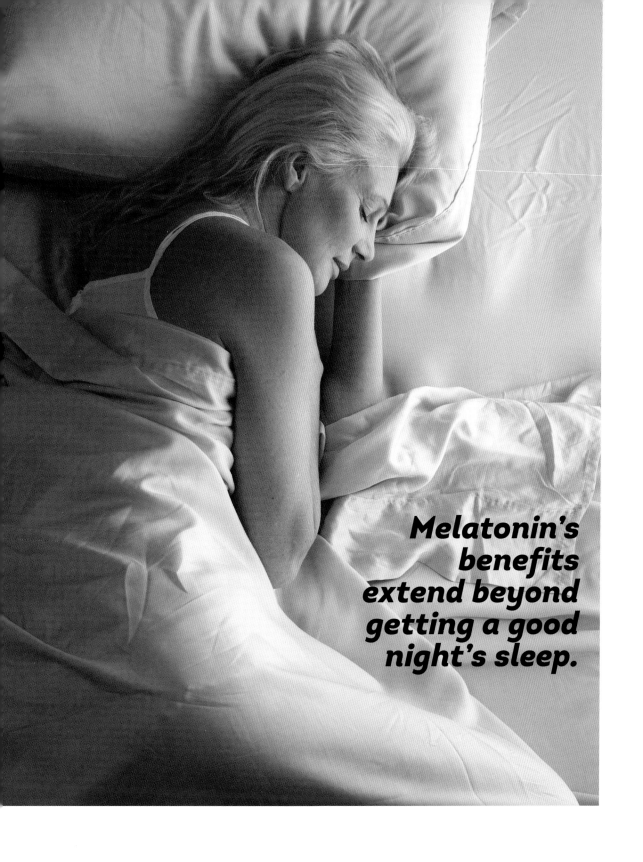

Melatonin's benefits extend beyond getting a good night's sleep.

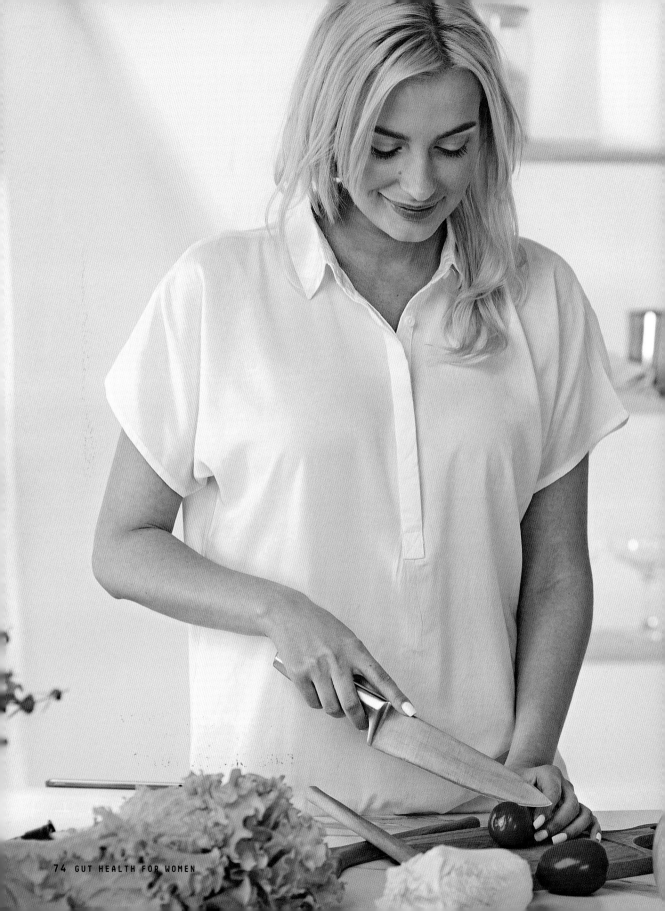

part

~

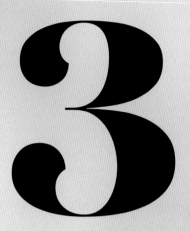

3

In the Kitchen

CHANGING UP YOUR DIET CAN GIVE YOU FRESH INSIGHT
INTO THE WAYS THE FOODS YOU'RE EATING AFFECT YOUR HEALTH.

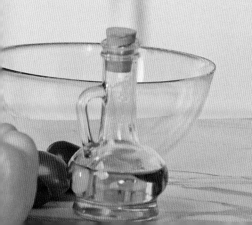

Eat Your Way Healthy

A STEP-BY-STEP PLAN TO FEELING BETTER

READY TO MAKE A CHANGE? THIS GUIDE WALKS YOU THROUGH HOW TO DO IT AND WHAT TO EXPECT.

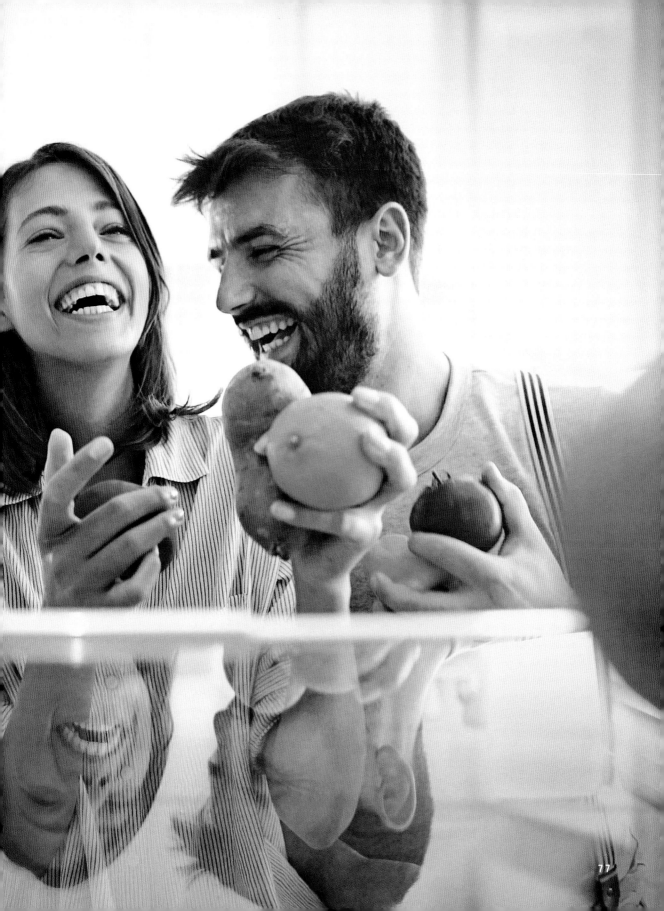

Stock Up

Gut expert Kitty Martone provides detailed weekly shopping lists in her book, as well as tips for prepping your kitchen. Some of the foods to stock up on:

- ✔ Almonds, raw
- ✔ Bay leaves
- ✔ Cashews
- ✔ Cayenne pepper
- ✔ Chia seeds
- ✔ Cinnamon
- ✔ Cumin
- ✔ Curry powder
- ✔ Flaxseed
- ✔ Garlic powder
- ✔ Ghee (clarified butter)
- ✔ Italian herb blend
- ✔ Lentils, beans
- ✔ Oats (gluten-free)
- ✔ Pumpkin seeds, raw
- ✔ Quinoa
- ✔ Vanilla extract
- ✔ Wild rice

At some point it happened: You turned into one of those people who has to be vigilant about what they eat for fear of feeling bloated, gassy, nauseous or just unwell. Your gut has become your Achilles' heel. "A lot of people come to me with other types of issues and they don't realize they're related to gut health," says Kitty Martone, author of *The 4-Week Gut Health Plan: 75 Recipes to Help Restore Your Gut* and host of the podcast Stuff Your Doctor Should Know. "The main problem, though, is discomfort after eating, whether that's bloating, gas or whatever."

Whether you're having digestion problems, other weird complaints, or just want to feel better, it may be time for a reset. You could try eating healthy, like following the Mediterranean diet (it's actually gut-healthy) or giving up alcohol and sugar, but to see how different foods may be contributing to your symptoms, consider a gut-focused 30-day plan. Why so long? Although you can see changes in the microbiome within 24 hours, during a four-week plan you can go a little deeper, says Martone. "It's a more intermediate level of upregulating digestion," she explains. "You're not just making better food choices; you're eliminating common allergens and foods that might be causing digestive distress." This is true whether you're following her plan, which she lays out in her book, or something like an elimination diet, Whole30 or the Autoimmune Protocol (AIP). Whichever diet you want to follow (gut-friendly or otherwise), here's how to make it through:

> **TIP**
> Always ask your doctor if there are any dietary changes you can make before you're given a drug.

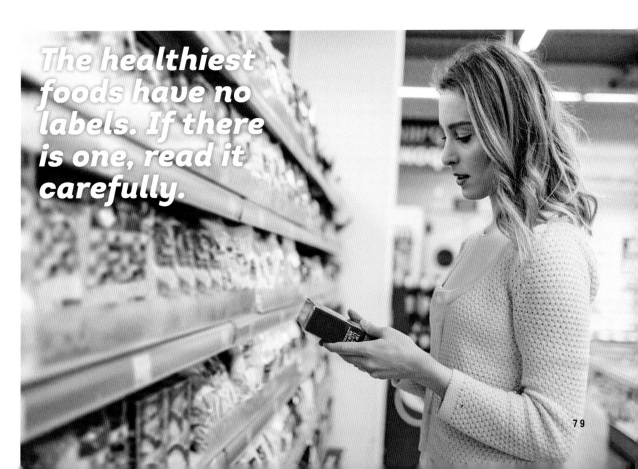

The healthiest foods have no labels. If there is one, read it carefully.

Step 1
Find the Right Plan for You

There are a variety of eating styles out there, whatever your goal. If you think you may be having an allergic reaction to food—you have pain, diarrhea, trouble breathing, itchiness or hives, or other significant symptoms after eating certain things—see a doctor before you try an elimination diet. (Obviously, severe symptoms warrant a trip to the ER.) If you just want to see how you can feel when you eat super clean, there's no need to check in with your physician. Consider your lifestyle (are you an athlete, for instance) and how you'll make this new way of eating fit in. (For a closer look at some of the more common gut-friendly diets out there and how they rate, turn to page 92.)

Step 2
Take Inventory of Your Pantry

Every diet is different, but all of them will require a shift to healthier eating—and that takes some prep, since you'll most likely be cooking more than you used to. "Organization is everything," says Martone. "Just as you would with an exercise goal, you need a plan, otherwise you're just floundering." First step: Get rid of any tempting foods you may already have around the house. Put them in the freezer, out of sight and/or reach, or just throw them out. Then go shopping and stock your pantry, fridge and freezer with everything you'll need to make healthy eating easy and convenient. (See page 78 for a starter list, and page 82 for foods to avoid.) If you need better kitchen tools (knives, food processors, slow cookers) to help you prepare all the healthy food, now's the time to invest.

Having a meal-prep day—many people do it on Sundays—will make it easy to stick with the eating plan during the week when you tend to be short on time. Go shopping, then arrange the foods so you can reach for them quickly: Chop veggies, cook stock, make or thaw sauces; you can then prepare complete meals and pop them in the freezer.

Planning is key when it comes to eating out, too. Restaurants can be a veritable minefield for anyone who's trying to eat in a healthy way or has some dietary restrictions. Make it easier on yourself by lobbying your dining companions for a venue that has healthy options and checking out the menu ahead of time.

Step 3
Adjust Your Mindset

Go into your meal plan with the intention to stick with whatever program you're doing, but don't be unforgiving of yourself if you have the occasional slip-up. "People put these limitations on themselves, and if they cheat in the first week or two, they beat themselves up," says Martone. "You can be strict without being mean to yourself, or angry if you mess up. It's not do-or-die." If you 'cheat' and have a cocktail or sandwich or whatever you're not supposed to have, vow to do better the next time you eat something and take it from there. The key is consistency, not rigidity.

Step 4
Find an Accountability Partner

Whether it's a significant other, friends, co-workers or an online community, having people to cheer you on is crucial for maintaining any new habit. Surround yourself with people who are encouraging —and let them know how you want to be supported. Some people bristle at questions about their diet; others are looking to share, and they want someone to call them out if they're slipping.

Step 5
Address Your Lifestyle

Diet certainly impacts gut health, but other lifestyle habits have very strong roles as well. Sleep, stress and exercise are all huge factors that can impact the microbiome on a daily basis. "The biggest mistake I see is people eating when they're totally stressed," says Martone. "Often that's part of the first complaint they have: They get bloated whether they eat a salad or a hamburger. Turns out they're in a hurry, they're on the go, they're eating when they're upset, eating fast and not chewing. It all has to do with being stressed-out while they eat."

Finding ways to manage stress—prayer or meditation, mindfulness, breath work, yoga, time with loved ones—will go a long way toward calming your nervous system and gut.

Step 6
Start Reintroducing Foods

If you've been following a more restrictive diet, most people usually start adding back foods into their regular meals after about a month or so. This is perhaps the most enlightening part of the whole endeavor, because it enables you to get evidence and really see how certain foods that you've now eliminated may wreak havoc on your system when you starting eating them again. Maybe you don't miss that gluten or those eggs or soy-based foods, and you don't want to add them back. No problem! But if you miss your sandwiches or yogurt, add them back in one at a time so you can pinpoint which item causes which symptoms. (A nutritionist can guide you in how much and how often to add food in, if you're not sure.)

What to Expect

Here's what gut expert Kitty Martone often sees happening with her clients when they first tackle a more restricted diet, such as the Autoimmune Protocol (AIP), keto or Whole30.

WEEK 1 You're generally eliminating foods here and settling into some new habits. You may not be feeling anything different except perhaps some low-level anxiety or stress about giving up some foods you're used to eating, and learning how to prepare new foods.

WEEK 2 Your microbiome is getting used to this new way of eating. You might notice your bowel movements changing; you might feel foggy-headed, tired or slightly feverish and achy. This is common in the second week, as your body is handling the detritus from various bugs or fungi dying off (it's called a die-off reaction, and it can even happen when you take prescription drugs), says Martone. Log what you're feeling in your food diary.

WEEK 3 You might feel excited about how you're feeling (no more headaches or bloating!) or start to notice things that tend to trip you up (happy hour, stressful events). You're troubleshooting here and making adjustments, says Martone. Have confidence that your body is changing, though!

WEEK 4 Like seedlings bursting through the soil in the springtime, you should be noticing some new shifts, whether it's a lack of GI complaints, better skin, or even improved sleep. Stay attuned to what's happening and be patient if the shift isn't as dramatic as you expected.

What to Eat
OR NOT

EVERY DIET IS DIFFERENT, BUT AUTHOR KITTY MARTONE KEEPS THE FOLLOWING FOODS ON HER RADAR DURING A GUT RESET. ONCE YOU'VE FIGURED OUT YOUR TRIGGERS YOU CAN ADJUST AS NECESSARY.

	Green Light	Yellow Light	Red Light
	Good for digestion, nutrition, gut healing, on or off a diet	*Choose in moderation (a few servings a week); they may trigger issues in some people*	*Avoid: They're poor in nutrition, highly processed and/or can cause inflammation*
	Coconut oil, ghee, cultured butter, olive oil, sesame oil	Butter, commercially processed oils	Imitation butter spreads, canola oil, corn oil, margarine, safflower or soy oil
	Kefir, goat cheese, nut milk	Cheese (hard, aged), yogurt (no sugar added)	Whipped cream, creamers, milk (nonorganic), sour cream, flavored yogurt
	Berries, green apples, lemons, limes	Red apples, bananas, dates	Juicing
	Arugula, asparagus, avocado, cauliflower, daikon, garlic, kale, potatoes, spinach, zucchini	Eggplant, peppers, potatoes (russet), tomatoes (these are nightshades)	Juicing

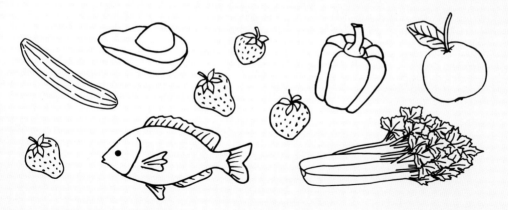

	Green Light *Good for digestion, nutrition, gut healing, on or off a diet*	**Yellow Light** *Choose in moderation (a few servings a week); they may trigger issues in some people*	**Red Light** *Avoid: They're poor in nutrition, highly processed and/or can cause inflammation*
	Brown rice, buckwheat, quinoa, spelt	Oats (gluten-free), popcorn, blue corn tortilla chips	Barley, bulgur, cereals, chips, cookies, pasta, white rice, wheat
	Organic, grass-fed beef/ bison, lamb; bone broths; organic free-range chicken, turkey and eggs	Commercially raised beef, lamb, pork, veal	Bacon, processed meats, sausage
	Oysters, scallops, squid, trout, wild-caught salmon and shrimp	Halibut, canned tuna, sea bass	Orange roughy, shark, swordfish
	Almonds, cashews, pecans, pistachios, walnuts	Raw beans (home-cooked)	Canned beans, roasted, salted nuts, peanuts and peanut butter, soybeans

BETTER DIGESTION FROM
A to Z

*NOT SURE WHAT TO EAT? THE FOLLOWING FOODS
(AND COMPOUNDS FOUND IN THEM) CAN HELP GUT HEALTH.
FROM APPLES TO ZUCCHINI, HERE'S WHAT TO
ADD TO YOUR SHOPPING LIST SO YOU CAN FEEL BETTER.*

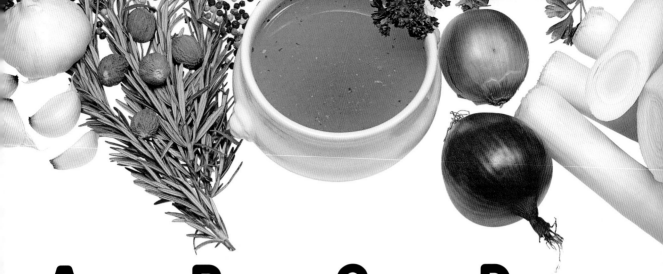

A Crunchy, naturally sweet **APPLES** are full of fiber, which helps feed good bugs in the gut, as well as polyphenols, plant compounds that have a variety of health benefits. Some research has suggested the polyphenols in apples may be able to help lower cholesterol. Be warned, though: There really are some "bad apples." Granny Smith, Red Delicious, Gala and Honey Crisp tend to have less sugar and more healthy compounds than other types. Buy organic to minimize pesticides—and keep the skin on, since that's where a big chunk of the nutrients are.

B **BONE BROTH** is the carnivore's celery juice, but with more health benefits. Rich in collagen, zinc and selenium, it's considered a health and joint tonic. The compounds in bone broth may also be able to help heal a leaky gut. (See page 162 for a recipe for chicken bone broth.)

Americans consume 20 pounds of apples per person a year.

C All sorts of research has documented the health effects of **CHOCOLATE**, especially dark varieties, and this may be why: Your gut bugs love it! As soon as it hits the large intestine, the bacteria pile on and the byproducts of the feasting may help fight inflammation in addition to lowering blood pressure, according to researchers from Louisiana State University. It helps keep the good bugs happy. Look for chocolate with a high cacao content (the higher it is, the more bitter it might taste) and a short list of ingredients.

D A cruciferous vegetable (they come packed with healthy plant power), the **DAIKON** radish is long, white and mildly spicy. It's excellent for digestion because it helps the body break down proteins and fats. Even daikon seeds are good for the gut. Often fermented, it's a common ingredient in kimchi, salads and soups and is an excellent addition to any heavy meal. Its plant compounds are purported to have anti-microbial and anti-cancer properties, among others. The leaves are edible as well, so you can use the entire vegetable.

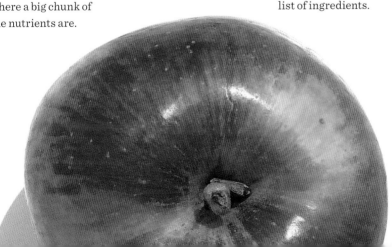

Honey doesn't boost blood sugar as much as table sugar.

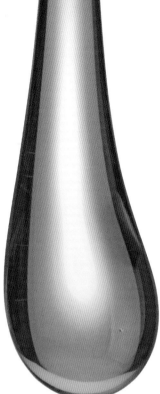

EGGS are packed with protein and other key nutrients, which make them a healthy breakfast staple. They can also be a quick, easy meal or snack at any time of the day. And they are relatively easy to digest compared to some other high-protein foods like meat and legumes, making them a good option for those with inflammatory bowel disease. However, eggs may be a food-allergy trigger, especially among children, which is why it may make sense to include them in an elimination diet.

F By now, you know that those good bugs in your belly feed on **FIBER**, which may be one of the reasons that eating a diet rich in fiber (25 grams a day for women and 38 for men) leads to so many wonderful health benefits including lowering cholesterol, regulating the bowels and controlling blood sugar, making it easier to lose weight, and more. You'll find it in fruits, vegetables, whole grains and legumes (chickpeas, lentils, beans and other foods). Fiber also helps bulk up stools and move them along.

G Thanks to gluten and the bias against carbs, **GRAINS** get a bad rap. However, whole grains are nutrient rock stars, containing fiber, protein, B vitamins, antioxidants and more. Study after study has shown consuming whole grains helps reduce the risk of a variety of diseases. Diets that limit wheat products may also alter the gut microbiota in unhealthy ways, inhibiting good bacteria and the body's ability to regulate the immune system. (Many people who think they have a gluten sensitivity really have an issue with compounds called FODMAPs, which are various carbohydrates found in a variety of healthy foods.) Brown rice, quinoa and amaranth are grains that tend to be easy on the digestion.

H Known to have antimicrobial and antioxidant properties, **HONEY** also functions as a prebiotic, meaning it helps feed healthy bacteria in the gut. It's not a license to go crazy with the sticky stuff, considering how sweet it is, but it can be used as a slightly healthier substitute to table sugar. Look for the "True Source Certified" logo on your honey, and shop farmers markets for honey produced locally, if possible.

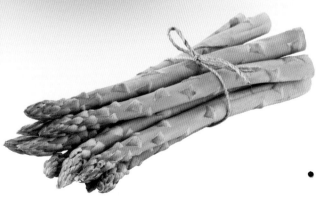

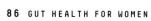

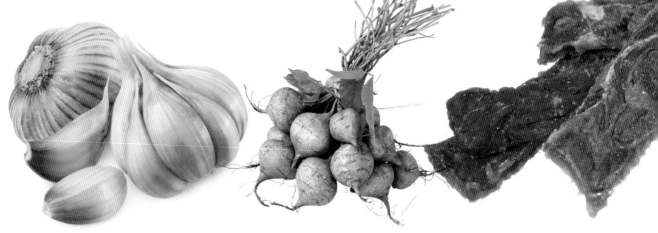

I Another prebiotic food, **INULIN** is a type of soluble fiber that occurs naturally, but it's also increasingly added to foods (think: bars, drinks and cereals) to boost the fiber content. Asparagus, onion, jicama and garlic contain inulin, but chicory root is the source for the inulin added to foods. Besides providing a smorgasbord for your good bugs, it also helps promote regular bowel habits and may help with weight loss. It's added to so many foods today that it's easy to get too much, which can lead to gut distress (gas, bloating, diarrhea). In addition, the more processed (ground-up) fiber is, the less effective it becomes.

J **JICAMA** (the "j" is pronounced like an "h"), a beige, starchy, bland-tasting legume, can be tossed into salads, slaws and stir-fries for some extra crunch, made into chips, and even eaten raw. It's high in vitamin C and soluble fiber (including inulin) and is a prebiotic food. It looks like a squat potato—but, being a member of the legume family, it boasts all sorts of healthy plant compounds, including antioxidants.

K Take green or black tea and add a little sugar, bacteria and yeast and you've got **KOMBUCHA** (aka "booch"), a fermented tea that's ubiquitous on store shelves. The fermentation process results in lactic acid bacteria that normally have a huge role in gut health, although whether they make it to the gut intact is still up for discussion. Kombucha retains all the healthy compounds of the tea it's made with, including antioxidant capabilities. Check the label for sugar content, as some commercially made drinks are high in sugar and calories.

L **L-GLUTAMINE** is an amino acid that the body creates naturally. Its spotlight role in the gut is in helping to repair the cells lining the digestive tract. (It can also help promote antioxidant and detoxification processes in the body.) You can find it naturally in foods—including beef, chicken, fish, eggs, dairy, legumes, cruciferous vegetables and beets—or take it in supplement form. People who have gut disorders like IBS, IBD, Crohn's and other issues sometimes take glutamine.

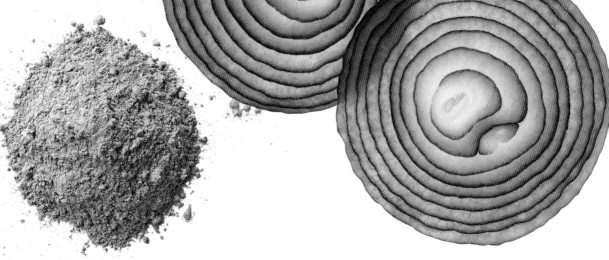

M An innocuous looking paste, **MISO** is made from fermenting soybeans with mold (mmm, yummy) and it's a chef's secret weapon. The salty, umami flavor provides depth and heft to dishes, from savory to sweet. You can use it to make soup, salad dressings and spreads, or even as an ingredient in baked goods. Thanks to the fermentation, it's considered a probiotic food that may help repopulate the good bugs in your gut. Look for it in the refrigerated foods section.

N Feeling adventurous? **NATTO**, fermented soybean, is a pungent, slimy, food that's rich in friendly bacteria that may help keep gut bugs balanced. It's not dissimilar to what happens when a leftover can of garbanzo beans gets too ripe in the fridge, although the fermentation process for natto is much more controlled. It's high in protein and fiber, natch. Bold eaters can dive in headfirst. If you're more skittish, add it to eggs, fried rice or anything that needs a little kick of flavor.

O There's a reason **ONIONS** are the base of so many different dishes. Besides providing flavor, they're a prebiotic food, so including them in your meal is like taking a little digestion and health booster. They also contain the polyphenol quercetin, which may have beneficial effects on the circulatory system (blood vessels) as well as the gut.

P You're better off getting your **PROBIOTICS** from foods like kimchi, sauerkraut, kefir and miso, but you can also look for them in supplement form. While research is still figuring out which bugs are best for the gut, and how best to deliver them to the nether regions of your digestive system intact, many experts recommend looking for a probiotic that contains 5 to 10 billion colony-forming units and a mélange of probiotic strains. Then change it up every few months.

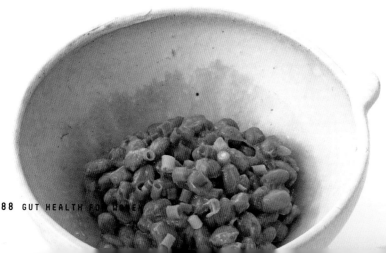

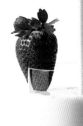

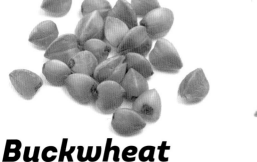

Buckwheat contains rutin and is high in fiber.

Q A relative of the apple and pear—both fiber-rich, good-for-you fruits—**QUINCE** is the way-lesser-known cousin. Hard to find (look for it in the fall) and not readily edible when raw, quince takes a little effort to prepare. Cooking it (roasting, baking or stewing) is the only way to truly release and enjoy its flavors. But it's high in vitamin C, polyphenols and a compound called pectin, which helps feed probiotics and contributes to a healthy gut lining.

R **RUTIN** is another plant polyphenol that has an impact in the digestive tract. A 2018 mouse study in *Frontiers In Microbiology* showed rutin, in combination with inulin, helped promote a healthy, diverse microbiome by keeping bad bugs in check, and also reduced inflammation. It's found in apples, tea, asparagus and other foods (which also often contain inulin).

S **SQUASH**— spaghetti, acorn, butternut and many more—is a staple for plant-based eaters. Its bright flesh is a sign that the vegetable is full of nutrients (including vitamins A and C) and certain types, such as acorn and butternut, are high in fiber. (One cup of acorn squash contains almost 10 grams of fiber!)

T **TEA**, which is high in antioxidants and other healthy plant compounds, has been around for centuries. It's often consumed with meals in various cultures, and there's a reason: The polyphenols in black tea, in particular, make a beeline (or tealine?) to your digestive tract, where the flavonols help support good gut bugs and soothe digestion. Herbal teas (technically called tisanes), such as chamomile or peppermint, may also help ease digestive symptoms like bloating or heartburn.

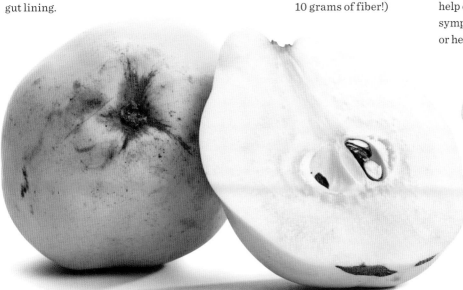

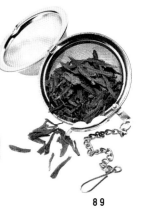

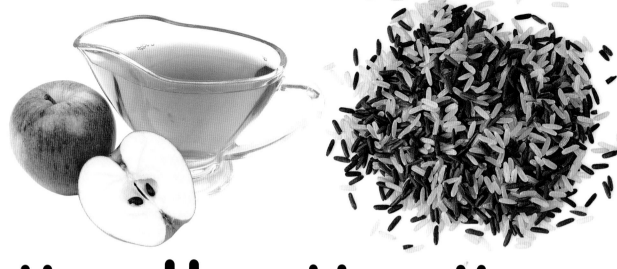

U Foods like natto and miso have an **UMAMI** flavor, a complex, savory, almost visceral taste that seems to satisfy taste buds far beyond your tongue. In fact, there appear to be receptors for the umami flavor in the gut. Monosodium glutamate, or MSG, in Asian cuisine is the classic umami flavor, but aged cheese, mushrooms and meat have it as well. (Cult-favorite ranch dressing is an umami bomb!) Researchers are studying this flavor as a way to stimulate appetite in the elderly. The taste comes from glutamate, an amino acid, which is important for stimulating digestion and maintaining a healthy gut lining.

V **VINEGAR,** especially apple cider vinegar, is revered in many gut-health circles. Its sour taste comes from the fermentation process and as a result, many people espouse drinking it, especially in the morning, as a health elixir. Research has shown vinegar may help control blood sugar and aid weight loss, in addition to having anti-bacterial properties, but note that chugging it on the regular can be hard on your teeth and esophagus. (Which means if you drink it, be sure to dilute.) Instead, use it in salad dressings and other dishes to add a little zing.

W **WILD RICE,** which is actually a seed, can be an excellent substitute for wheat if you're sensitive or intolerant, and it's a more nutritious alternative to white rice. One cup contains almost 3 grams of fiber and 6 grams of protein. A much-cited *Journal of Agricultural and Food Chemistry* study found it contains 30 times more antioxidants than white rice. It's also versatile, in that you can add it to other dishes instead of just eating it on its own.

X A sugar-free sweetener, **XYLITOL** comes from a plant and is commonly added to gum, candy and other products to reduce the calorie count while still preserving sweetness. This prebiotic can offer some benefits for your gut while reducing sugar intake, but beware of high doses, which can cause gas, bloating and general discomfort.

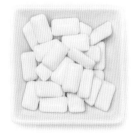

A cup of zucchini has just 20 calories. Pasta has about 200.

~

Y Another probiotic food, **YOGURT** is created by fermenting milk with two types of bacteria (Streptococcus thermophilus and Lactobacillus bulgaricus). Their byproducts are what result in that sour taste. Look for yogurt that contains "live, active cultures" and choose plain versus flavored, which often contains high amounts of sugar or sugar substitutes. (Some of the sugar in yogurt comes naturally from the milk.) You can choose plant-based yogurts if the milk bothers your digestion. Bonus: A *New England Journal of Medicine* study found that people who eat yogurt regularly have an easier time controlling their weight.

Z In these post-kale times, **ZUCCHINI** is riding high, thanks to the invention of the spiralizer, a handy gadget that takes a boring old summer squash and turns it into fun ribbons that you can use in place of pasta for a low-cal, equally tasty dish. It's high in water and fiber—goodbye constipation—and boasts potassium and B vitamins among other healthy plant compounds.

~
Got tummy
troubles? Start
with diet.

WHICH
Gut Diet
IS BEST?

THERE IS A VARIETY OF WAYS TO TACKLE GI ISSUES,
BUT THEY'RE NOT ALL EASY TO FOLLOW.

I f you're having digestive trouble—gas, bloating, constipation, upset stomach—the standard advice you're most likely to get is to: 1) eat more fiber; or 2) watch your diet. But where do you go from there? And when the symptoms go *beyond* the GI tract—brain fog, headaches, achy joints, acne—it's likely your diet will never even come up at a doctor's visit. Most physicians aren't trained in nutrition and don't refer you to a nutritionist to help you wade through the many options out there.

Besides, the standard diet advice isn't always helpful for gut issues. Yes, it might help you lower your cholesterol or blood sugar, but the gastrointestinal tract is tricky. Every body is different and reacts to foods in its own way.

While in rare cases some of these symptoms can be signaling a serious problem, the majority of the time they aren't. A little sleuthing to suss out which foods are causing you trouble can save you money and help you avoid taking drugs that you don't need. If diet doesn't work, that's helpful information for your doc.

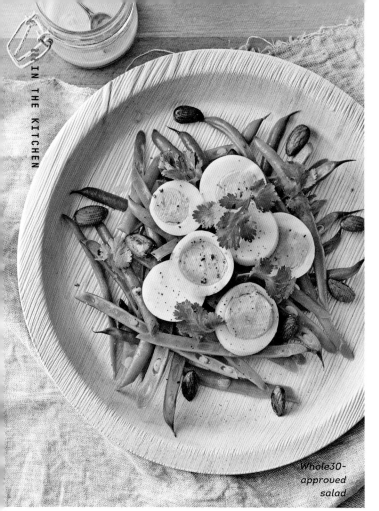

Whole30-approved salad

associated with health promotion and disease prevention....” Many of these diets are successful for weight loss because they restrict the foods you can eat—often to a point where you feel deprived.

Following are some of most popular diets that people use to “clean up” their eating and start anew. Most are meant to be a short-term solution, since they are restrictive and some, like the low-FODMAPs diet, temporarily cut out foods that, besides their tendency to promote gas and bloating, are otherwise very healthy and high in fiber. The ultimate goal is to find the way of eating that works best for *you*.

Elimination Diet

HOW IT WORKS Most of the diets here fall under the elimination umbrella in some way, but the traditional elimination diet is one that takes out those foods that are most likely to trigger an allergic reaction. (An allergic reaction will happen every time you eat the food, whereas a sensitivity might only happen on occasion, depending on how much of the food you eat.) If you truly think you’re allergic to a food, it’s important to check in with your doctor *before* you start a diet, while you’re still having symptoms. “You first need to identify whether your symptoms are being caused by your immune system or your digestive system,” says Julie Stefanski, RDN, a spokeswoman for the Academy of Nutrition and Dietetics who is in private practice in York, Pennsylvania. A physician can help you do that.

“It’s likely you’d start by eliminating one of the eight major allergens, which are soy, cow’s milk, tree nuts, peanuts, wheat, fish, shellfish and eggs,” she says. “They cause most of the allergic reactions in Americans.” You might also experiment with cutting out gluten,

If you’re looking to lose weight or cut out the junk, these diets may help as well, although many of them aren’t designed to be followed for the long term. A 2014 literature review published in the *Annual Review of Public Health* looked at research on a variety of diets and concluded: “Claims for the established superiority of any one specific diet over others are exaggerated. The weight of evidence strongly supports a theme of healthful eating while allowing for variations on that theme. A diet of minimally processed foods close to nature, predominantly plants, is decisively

TIP
Go to eatright.org to find a dietitian with gut smarts.

meat, sugar, alcohol, caffeine and other things to see what might be bothering your system, but these would usually be food sensitivities rather than allergies. You follow an elimination diet for three to four weeks and then slowly start adding back foods. (Nutritionists are uniquely qualified to help you manage this phase.)

PROS It's relatively quick and straightforward, and can be very enlightening.

CONS It can be restrictive, especially if you love your dairy, nuts or eggs. The more foods you cut out, the more restrictive it is, and the more time-consuming it can be to figuring out which is the offending item.

Mediterranean Diet

HOW IT WORKS This extremely well-researched diet—which is really more of an eating pattern—has earned kudos for its healthy, balanced approach. It emphasizes vegetables, whole grains, fruits, legumes, nuts, herbs and spices, seafood and healthy fats. While it's not considered an elimination diet, it's still very good for gut health, since it's high in fiber and eschews processed, sugary foods. Recent research, published in the journal *Gut*, found that this way of eating reduced inflammation and preserved beneficial gut bacteria associated with brain function in the elderly.

PROS If you're not very good at restriction, this may be the best "diet" to start with. This is a plan you can easily stick with in the long term.

CONS There are very few, but one is that it doesn't eliminate any food—besides junk—that might cause sensitivities (like FODMAPs), so it may not help you ID triggering foods.

Whole30

HOW IT WORKS This 30-day plan cuts out alcohol as well as soy, grains (whole and processed), sugar and legumes. Meat,

vegetables, healthy fats and limited fruits are all on the "green light" list. Once the diet ends, you can add back in the foods you enjoy and you'll be much more aware of how those foods make you feel.

PROS There's no cabbage soup or other gimmicks or craziness here, and if you're addicted to sugar, in whatever form, this plan can help you kick the habit. There are a handful of Whole30–branded cookbooks out there to help you get through the initial diet and beyond.

CONS It's restrictive. The limitation on grains and legumes is unfortunate, but it's only for 30 days.

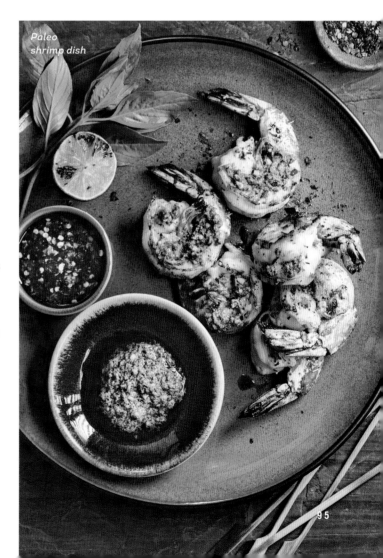

Paleo shrimp dish

Autoimmune Protocol (AIP)

HOW IT WORKS The typical Paleo (as in Paleolithic) diet is based on how humans used to eat back before we had access to tons of different types of food. It assumes that our genetics haven't adapted and changed over 10,000 years. It's heavy on lean meat, seafood, vegetables, fruits and nuts, and oils from these items (such as avocado, coconut or olive oil). It puts the kibosh on dairy, legumes and grains, alcohol and, of course, anything processed or high in sugar. The AIP diet is an even more restrictive version of Paleo and is designed to cut out any potentially inflammatory foods. It also nixes eggs and nightshades (tomatoes, potatoes, eggplant and peppers), which some people may be sensitive to. You follow it for a month (or longer) and then start adding foods back in.

PROS "Taking out these foods is potentially helpful to heal the gut and the hope is that eventually you'll be able to tolerate these foods again," says Carley Smith, NTP, a nutritional therapist and creator of the Fairy Gutmother blog. "It may help reverse or lessen an autoimmune condition."

CONS It's restrictive and not meant to be followed long-term. There are more tolerable anti-inflammatory diets.

Keto

HOW IT WORKS Short for ketogenic, the keto diet is all about fat. It severely limits carbohydrates, with the hope that this will force the body to rely on (and get better at using) fat stores for energy. "Ketones, a metabolic byproduct of this way of eating, are thought to be a fuel source for some of the cells in the large intestine," says Smith.

PROS There is some interesting research on this diet, especially as it relates to people with

TIP
Keep a food diary to track your symptoms after eating.

seizures, diabetes and other health issues. Macronutrient ratios vary, from 60 to 75 percent fat, 20 to 35 percent protein and only about 5 to 10 percent carbohydrates.

CONS It's very restrictive and can be difficult to follow. "You're not getting the fiber that the gut needs to promote short-chain fatty acid production," says Smith. "But some research is showing the gut may be able to do it in a different way."

Low-FODMAPs Diet

HOW IT WORKS FODMAPs stands for fermentable oligosaccharides, disaccharides, monosaccharides and polyols. Many foods we think of as being healthy (including apples, milk, wheat, cherries and cauliflower) contain certain carbohydrates that are poorly absorbed in the intestines. They ferment, which causes gas, bloating and possibly diarrhea and abdominal pain.

You cut out foods that are high in FODMAPs in favor of foods that are low or moderate in content. Because so many offenders are very healthy, you don't want to be on this diet for a long time. Usually, you follow it for several weeks and then add back foods.

PROS The cutting-out and adding-back phases make it relatively easy to figure out what's causing a problem.

CONS It can be restrictive.

GAPS DIET

HOW IT WORKS Developed by Natasha Campbell-McBride, MD, the GAPS (Gut and Psychology Syndrome) diet was initially developed as a way to treat people with neurological or mental/emotional conditions, such as autism spectrum disorder and ADD/ADHD. The thinking is that what happens in the gut is affecting the brain (see page 34

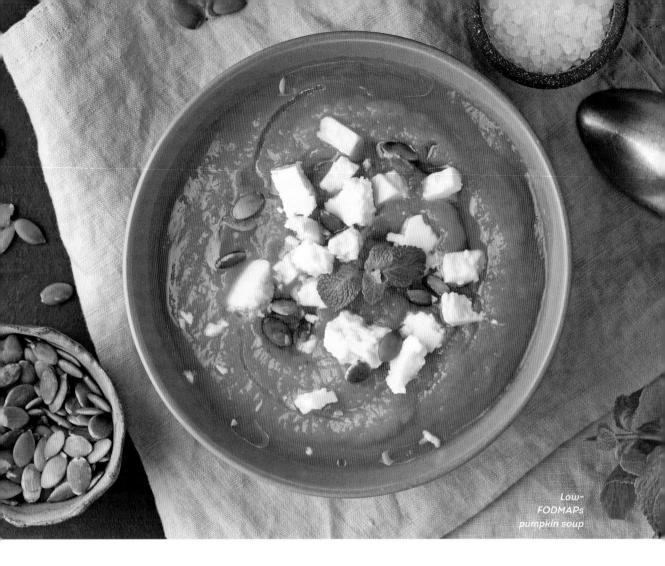

Low-FODMAPs pumpkin soup

for more on that). It involves different stages designed to help you detox from what you were eating before, restore a healthy balance of gut bugs, and then heal the gut lining. "You're supposed to be on it for two years maximum, but most people don't do that," says Smith. Some people skip the painful introductory phase and go straight to the full diet, which is more sustainable.

The introductory phase of the GAPS diet includes drinking lots of bone broth (to heal the gut lining) and eating probiotic foods. The full diet allows you to have meat, eggs, some vegetables, certain fermented foods and seafood. Fruits, sugars and processed foods aren't allowed. Eventually, the goal is to add a variety of foods back in, and be able to tolerate them.

PROS People who are suffering from chronic issues that are not responding to drugs or other treatment may be willing to try such a longer-term, restrictive diet. If this is the only thing that can help, it's worth it. A GAPS practitioner can help you dial in what might work best for you. (Find one at gaps.me.)

CONS The diet can be very difficult to follow, and it hasn't been studied extensively.

the ABCs of a FODMAPs diet

THIS ODD-SOUNDING EATING APPROACH IS A KEY TOOL FOR GETTING TO THE ROOT OF DIGESTIVE TROUBLES.

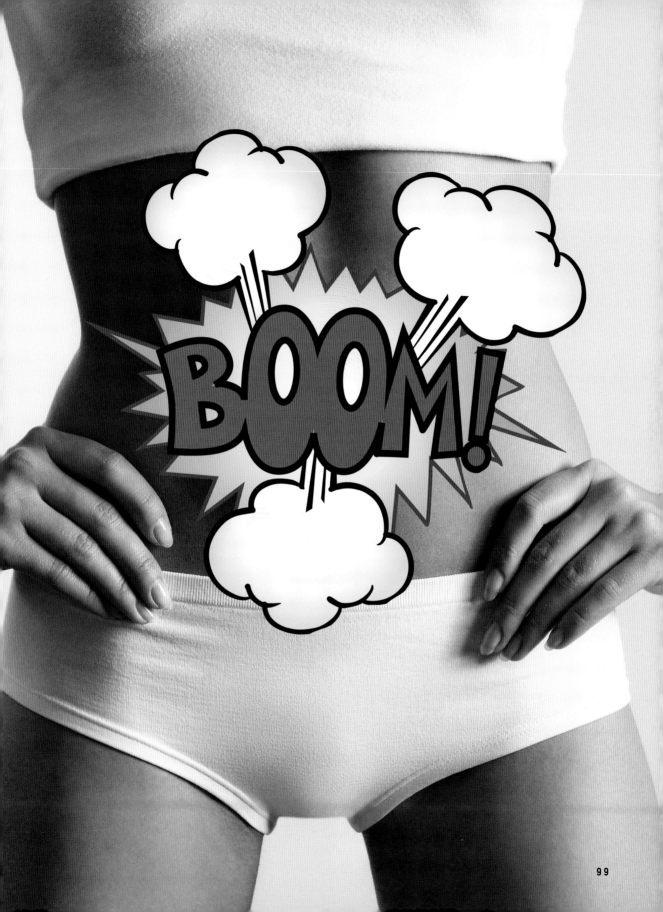

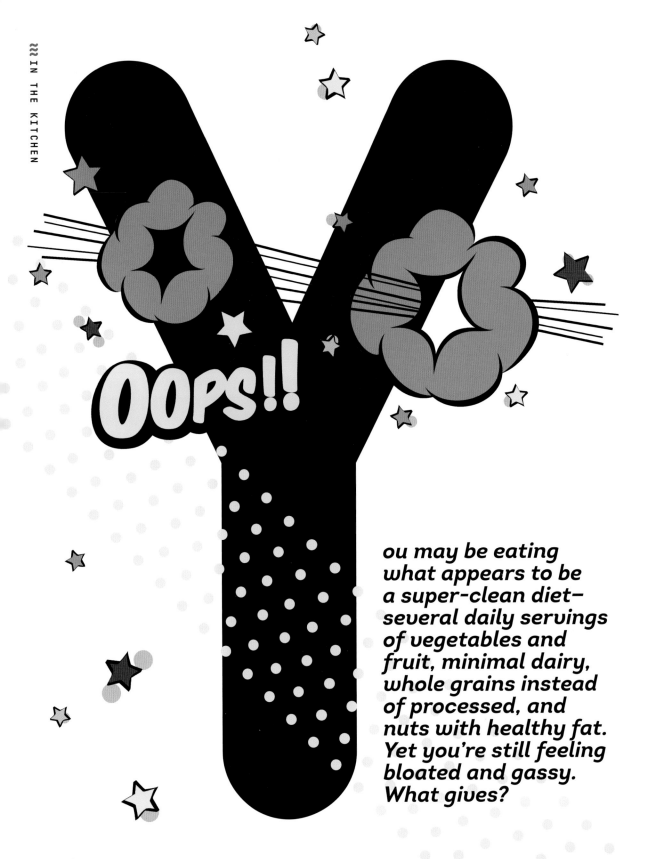

OOPs!!

ou may be eating what appears to be a super-clean diet— several daily servings of vegetables and fruit, minimal dairy, whole grains instead of processed, and nuts with healthy fat. Yet you're still feeling bloated and gassy. What gives?

Many healthy foods contain certain types of carbohydrates that are poorly absorbed in the intestines. As a result, they sit in the gut where they ferment, thanks to bacteria. It's the waste products from these bugs that lead to gas, bloating and sometimes diarrhea and abdominal pain. Dubbed FODMAPs—which stands for fermentable oligosaccharides, disaccharides, monosaccharides and polyols—these short-chain carbohydrates (common in high-fiber foods) can be powerful triggers of digestive symptoms. Sometimes it's something as simple as lactose, the sugar in cow's milk, or fructose, the sugar in fruit, that's the culprit, but other times it's more complicated.

"We use the FODMAPs diet every day in some capacity," says Melissa Phillips, RDN, a clinical nutritionist with the University of Wisconsin Health System's Digestive Health Center in Madison. "We've found that it does help a fairly significant number of patients when it's done correctly, with dietitian-led nutrition counseling and follow-up. It allows people to find their triggers and manage them, as well as expand their diet in terms of foods that don't cause symptoms." (Turns out, gluten sensitivity may actually be due to the FODMAPs in certain grains and not gluten itself.)

Research has shown that following a low-FODMAPs diet (low, not zero) can relieve symptoms of irritable bowel syndrome, or IBS—one of the most common gastrointestinal disorders—especially when there's abdominal pain involved, says Meagan Bridges, RD, a clinical dietitian at the University of Virginia Health System. "The FODMAPs effect varies. It tends to help more people with diarrhea than constipation, but it also tends to help people who have either one when it's accompanied by abdominal pain and discomfort." (Researchers

Breaking Down the FODMAPs

Carbohydrates are just sugar molecules linked in chains. The FODMAPs carbs are known as short-chain carbohydrates, meaning they have 10 or fewer sugars on the molecule, and they may sound familiar.

OLIGOSACCHARIDES
Most people can't break down these common carbohydrates, but people with IBS may be more sensitive to them than others. Onions, chicory root, Jerusalem artichokes, wheat, garlic and many other foods contain oligosaccharides.

DISACCHARIDES Lactose, found in milk products, is a disaccharide, and it's a common cause of digestive problems in people who lack sufficient amounts of the dietary enzyme lactase, which aids absorption of lactose.

MONOSACCHARIDES Also known as simple sugars, monosaccharides include glucose, fructose and galactose. Fructose is the naturally occurring sugar found in fruit, as well as honey, agave and high-fructose corn syrup. According to the International Foundation of Gastrointestinal Disorders, 30 to 40 percent of healthy people have difficulty absorbing excess amounts of fructose.

POLYOLS Sugar alcohols are used as sugar substitutes. Some, such as sorbitol and mannitol, are also found in certain medications.

believe the pain comes from excess water being released into the small intestine during digestion, which may contribute to diarrhea and abdominal symptoms. The fermentation process in the large intestine also leads to lots of gassy bacteria and that gas accumulates in the large intestine, causing discomfort.)

A 2016 research review in the journal *Clinical and Experimental Gastroenterology* showed that a low-FODMAPs diet is better at relieving IBS symptoms than the standard "healthy eating advice" to adjust fiber intake and avoid sugar and sugar alcohols. Some research has shown this type of diet also helps people with Crohn's disease and ulcerative colitis.

Finding Your Happy-Belly Place

Although you can easily Google lists of high- and low-FODMAPs foods (or see page 104) and start cutting out suspected offenders, Phillips notes that it's not a diet to follow in the long term, especially since there are so many healthy foods that are high in FODMAPs, including cherries, cauliflower, lentils and almonds. "It's meant to be a learning diet. Typically you follow it for several weeks and then start bringing back in individual foods over a three-day period to see how much, if any, you can eat before your symptoms start showing up." Working with a nutrition expert can help you more easily zero in on trigger foods and ensure that you're still getting plenty of healthy fiber and other nutrients in the interim. A dietitian can also help you slowly add back in higher-FODMAPs foods to find the "dose" that works best for you.

Note that prebiotics—those certain fiber-rich foods that help nourish your gut-bug population—are often high in FODMAPs. That's all the more reason to zero in on the specific foods that cause symptoms and identify alternatives you can consume.

Will the Ideal Gut-Friendly Diet Please Stand Up?

Bodies are weird. A diet that works for one person may not work for another. While there has been plenty of research about the ideal diet for heart health (kudos to the Mediterranean diet), the same hasn't happened yet for gut health. Keto (which emphasizes fats) and Paleo (which emphasizes vegetables, meat, fish and some nuts and restricts dairy, many grains, beans and lentils) diets often have good results when it comes to weight loss because you tend to eat fewer calories in general on them. While that can help some gut symptoms, it doesn't make them ideal.

"I think they both have gut-healthy components—but both of them also emphasize fats and animal proteins," says nutritional therapist Carley Smith, NTP, creator of the Fairy Gutmother blog. "Research shows that excess amounts of these can decrease the good bacteria in the gut, leading to inflammation. It's important to have a balanced diet with moderate amounts of sustainable proteins and healthy fats while at the same time incorporating plenty of fiber-rich foods to feed the beneficial bacteria. Grains and legumes, healthy sources of fiber, are often restricted in Paleo and keto diets, starving the beneficial bacteria."

These diets may also include high-FODMAPs foods (especially Paleo). If those are triggering symptoms, you'll have to suss out the culprits.

More than 30 studies have shown a low-FODMAPs diet can reduce IBS symptoms.

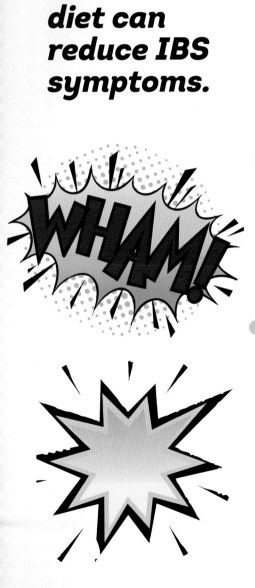

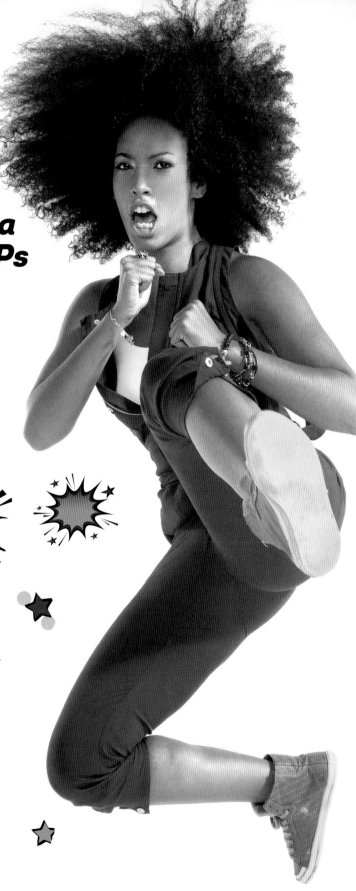

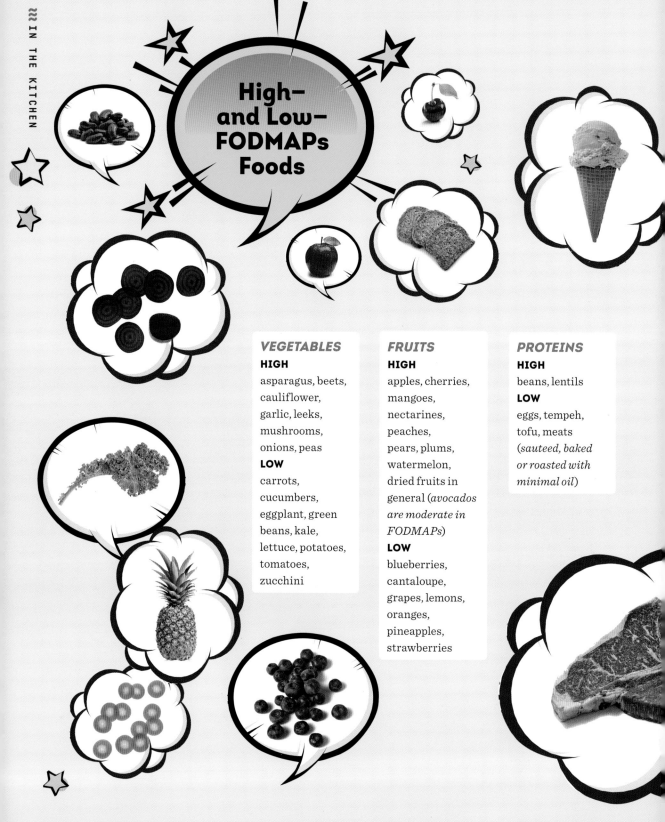

High– and Low–FODMAPs Foods

VEGETABLES

HIGH

asparagus, beets, cauliflower, garlic, leeks, mushrooms, onions, peas

LOW

carrots, cucumbers, eggplant, green beans, kale, lettuce, potatoes, tomatoes, zucchini

FRUITS

HIGH

apples, cherries, mangoes, nectarines, peaches, pears, plums, watermelon, dried fruits in general (*avocados are moderate in FODMAPs*)

LOW

blueberries, cantaloupe, grapes, lemons, oranges, pineapples, strawberries

PROTEINS

HIGH

beans, lentils

LOW

eggs, tempeh, tofu, meats (*sauteed, baked or roasted with minimal oil*)

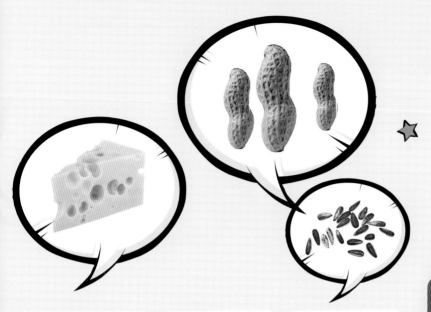

DAIRY

HIGH

cow's milk *(unless it's lactose-free)*, cream cheese, ice cream, sour cream, soy milk *(made from soy beans)*, yogurt

LOW

almond milk, butter, cottage cheese, feta cheese, hard cheeses

GRAINS

HIGH

wheat, rye, barley *(and products made with these)*

LOW

corn, oats, quinoa, rice *(and products made with these)*

NUTS & SEEDS

HIGH

almonds, cashews, hazelnuts, pistachios, sesame seeds, sunflower seeds

LOW

Brazil nuts, chia seeds, flaxseed, macadamia nuts, peanuts, pecans, pumpkin seeds, walnuts

Generally Safe Foods

Most oils except soybean; meat, poultry and seafood (prepared without sauces); maple syrup; table sugar (honey, agave and high-fructose corn syrup are high in FODMAPs)

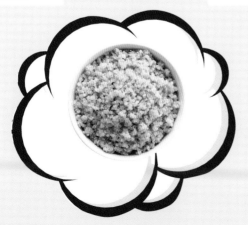

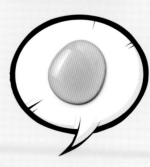

THE RIGHT WAY TO DO A
Cleanse

CELERY JUICE? CABBAGE SOUP? NOPE. HERE'S HOW TO HIT THE "RESET" BUTTON IN A HEALTHY WAY.

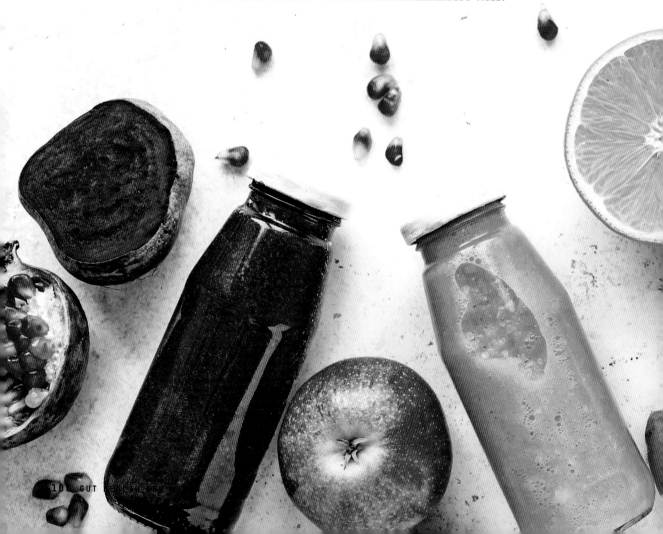

T he number of fad cleanses and "detox" diets can be overwhelming. It seems like new ones are always popping up—from juice and bone-broth regimens to supplements and super-restrictive diets. There are cleanses for your colon and liver, and detox kits for weight loss or an energy boost. But how many of these are effective— and moreover, since the body is fully capable of cleansing and detoxifying itself, are these regimens necessary?

X Marks the Toxin

First, you have to know what a toxin is. We're constantly bombarded with "toxins" in everyday life, from environmental assailants like pollutants, heavy metals and chemicals, to pesticides, to additives that are found in many of the foods we eat. The body generally does a great job of getting rid of things that aren't supposed to be there, because it's innately equipped with highly intelligent organs—like the lungs, liver, kidneys and colon, to name a few—that are constantly removing toxins. With

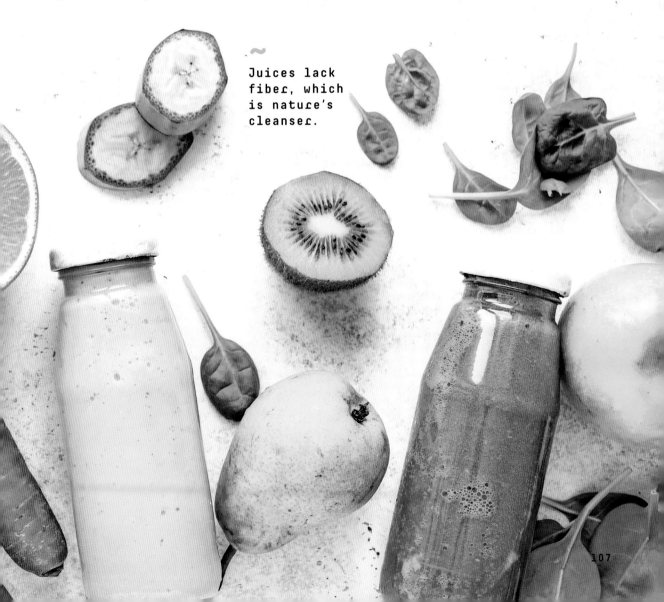

Juices lack fiber, which is nature's cleanser.

every bead of sweat and breath of air, the human body is systematically maintaining homeostasis, or balance. The lungs, for instance, filter toxins through bodily functions like coughing and sneezing. Even breathing is an act of cleansing, as you inhale oxygen that is transported to the blood and exhale carbon dioxide. The liver breaks down fats, excess amino acids (or proteins) and toxins in the blood and converts waste into urea, which is transported to the kidneys. These potato-size organs act as sieves, filtering blood and fluids and sending waste, or urine, to the bladder for removal. Finally, the colon absorbs water and carries waste solids from digestion, aka poop, out of the body.

A cleanse is typically a short-term therapy to help you eliminate toxins. It's used to stimulate the natural detoxification pathways and promote the elimination of contaminants. But rather than investing hundreds of dollars in trendy juices and supplements, try the best detox of all: removing processed foods and sugar from your diet. It's not so much a "detox" as a reset, avoiding harmful substances while incorporating foods that help support the body's innate detoxification system.

The Best Detox

Since the gut is home to one of the most significant "cleansing" systems in the body, the best way to support and reset it is by focusing on foods that enhance the microbiome and make waste removal, which naturally cleanses the body, easier. A healthy colon contains beneficial bacteria and fungi, as well as an intact gut lining. When there is an overgrowth of pathogenic organisms in the gut (you can think of them as toxins), it can cause the gut lining to become weak and permeable, allowing bad bugs to seep into the system; this can lead to inflammation (for more on what's commonly referred to as "leaky gut," turn to page 28).

According to Mahmoud Ghannoum, PhD, director of the Center for Medical Mycology at Case Western Reserve University, the foods you consume either support this optimal balance or contribute to an imbalance, leading to an overgrowth of pathogens like Candida and E. coli. It's critical to avoid refined sugars and starches in order to reduce fungal pathogens like Candida, because fungus thrives on sugar. At the same time, he says, "You must also support the beneficial

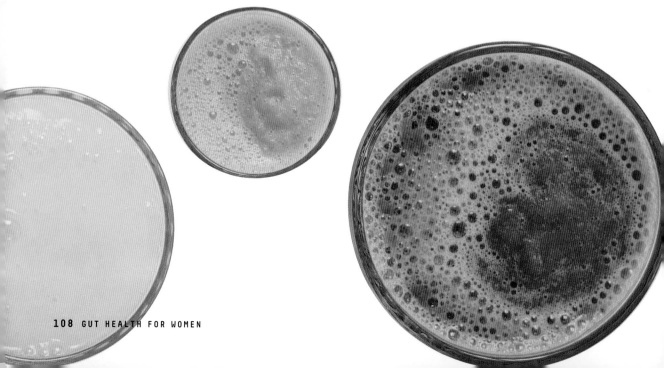

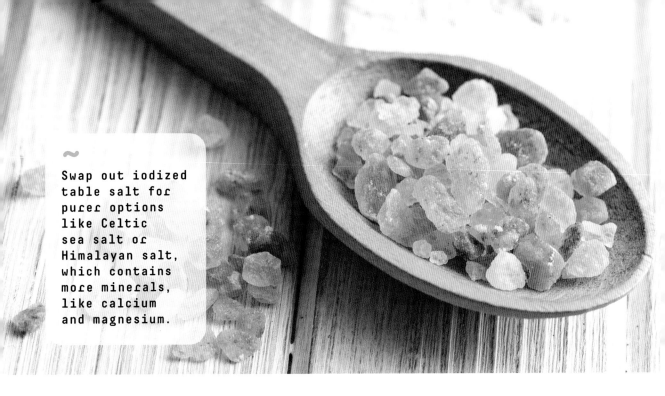

~

Swap out iodized table salt for purer options like Celtic sea salt or Himalayan salt, which contains more minerals, like calcium and magnesium.

organisms by incorporating foods rich in vitamins, as research shows deficiencies in vitamins A, B and C are correlated to fungal overgrowth." The good news, Ghannoum adds, is that fungi are rapidly changing molecules, and the microbiome can shift within 24 hours after dietary changes.

Fiber is one of the best foods for supporting the colon, because it helps feed the beneficial organisms in the gut, promoting optimal microbial balance. In addition to acting as food for the friendly microbes, it also helps encourage healthy and regular bowel movements by bulking up the stools, making them easier to pass. Without regular bowel movements (ideally at least once a day, although everyone is different), waste products begin to accumulate in the colon. This not only inhibits the body's ability to detoxify itself, but also throws off the microbial balance, causing additional health concerns.

TIP
"Addicted" to coffee? You may need a caffeine reset, too.

According to a 2019 study published in the *Journal of Probiotics and Health*, increasing fiber intake—as part of a 28-day, gut-health program called the Mycobiome Diet—led to a significant decrease in pathogens while promoting the growth and sustainability of beneficial organisms like Lactobacillus, a key species in fighting inflammation and promoting a strong immune system.

The research also states the best sources of fiber are resistant starches, which are literally just that: resistant to digestion, and instead break down or ferment in the large intestine by becoming snacks for the beneficial bacteria. Foods like whole grains, oats and potatoes are all excellent examples of resistant starches. Cruciferous vegetables like broccoli, cauliflower and cabbage, and leafy greens, are other sources of the fiber that supports optimal gut function. In addition to fiber, healthy fats and proteins are other important parts of microbial health.

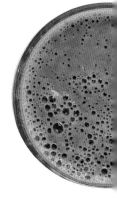

DIY 21-Day Cleanse

If you're looking for a simple and clean diet reset, try this three-week plan, including these specific dietary changes that help support a thriving microbiome. Although the gut can change in as few as 24 hours, allowing a few weeks not only helps ensure that optimal shifts in the microbiome have taken place, but it also gives the body time to eliminate any accumulated toxins. Essentially, for three weeks you will remove foods that have been known to negatively impact the gut—processed foods, sugar—and incorporate nutrient-dense foods that feed a healthy microbiome.

Foods to Incorporate Daily

>4 SERVINGS OF PROTEIN, ideally plant-based (serving sizes are in parentheses)
Legumes (beans, peas, lentils, peanuts) (1/2 cup cooked)
Nuts and seeds (1/4 cup)
Soy (edamame, tempeh, tofu) (4 ounces)
Grains (amaranth, quinoa, brown rice, teff) (1/2 cup cooked)
Animal-based chicken, fish, grass-fed beef, pasture-raised pork, bison (4 ounces)
Dairy aged cheeses like Parmesan, feta and Swiss (2 ounces), milk (8 ounces), plain yogurt (6 ounces)

> 4 SERVINGS OF FAT/OIL (1 to 2 tablespoons) Healthy cooking fats like ghee (clarified butter), coconut oil and grass-fed butter are excellent healthy fats, especially for all your high-temperature cooking and frying. Olive oil and avocado oil are great for salads or light sauteing.
> 3–6 SERVINGS OF RESISTANT STARCH Legumes, oats, potatoes, winter squash, underripe bananas
> 3 CUPS (minimum) VEGETABLES
All veggies and leafy greens

Foods to Eliminate

Processed/refined products
Crackers, frozen dinners, packaged meals, soups, condiments, dressing—all of these usually have tons of sodium, sugar, additives, preservatives and more. A quick rule of thumb: Opt for foods with fewer than five ingredients, because they are less likely to be processed.
Sugar (except for honey or maple syrup, used sparingly) Sugar hides out in packaged foods. A few commonly used sugar substitutes, which you should also avoid, are maltodextrin, corn syrup and sucralose, aka Splenda (there are dozens of names for sugar on food labels). Stick to more natural sweeteners like honey, which has anti-microbial and anti-inflammatory properties.

Alcohol Alcohol decreases microbial diversity in the gut and should be eliminated during the gut reset.

What About?

Coffee You can have coffee, preferably organic to ensure fewer pesticides and chemicals, ultimately yielding a more gut-friendly beverage.
Fruits Fruit is an excellent snack or dessert. Berries in particular are high in polyphenols, plant compounds that may be able to disrupt biofilms (see page 14).

After a week, or even a few days, on the diet, you may start to notice a shift in how your body feels. This can be unpleasant at first, like excess gas and bloating, which is totally normal (and actually a good sign!). It means the bacteria are starting to react to the increase in fiber, and by the second or third week these symptoms should subside as the gut adjusts. To mitigate these side effects, you can always try cooking your foods, which can make them easier to digest, and drink bone broth to ease stomach discomfort.

After 21 days, you should notice improved sleep patterns and an increase in energy levels. You may even notice you've lost a few pounds. You may have forgotten what feeling good feels like, but this is how your body is designed to function. You just have to give it the right support.

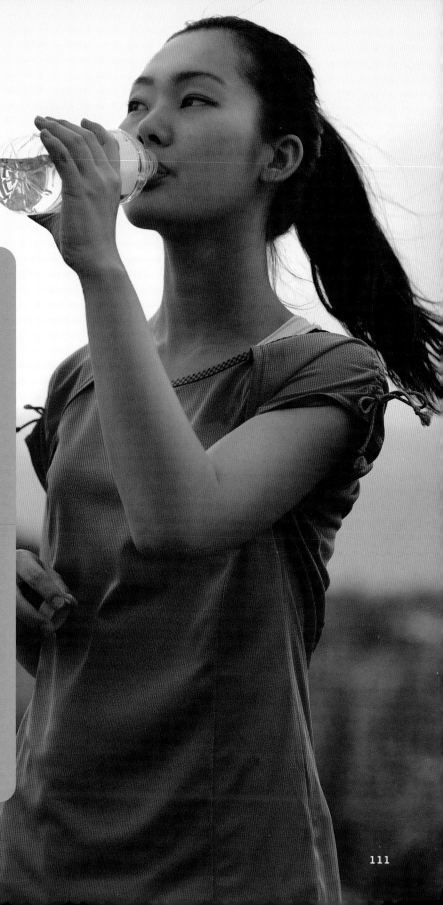

Take Your Detox a Step Further

Why stop at food when you're trying to feel better?

STAY HYDRATED *There are no hard-and-fast rules about how much water to drink, but you should be downing enough so that when you pee, it's pale yellow and not smelly. If you're hydrated, you're helping your kidneys flush everything out.*

WORK UP A SWEAT *While you can sweat out toxins, it won't make a huge difference. Instead, exercise helps improve your mood (not to mention overall health), and may boost bowel regularity, too.*

DO A TECH CLEANSE *Reducing screen time and social media scrolling can help reset your brain and improve your attention span. You may find that you have a more positive attitude and are less likely to feel depressed.*

CUT THE DEAD WEIGHT *Have negative people in your life? Cutting ties may make you feel lighter and happier.*

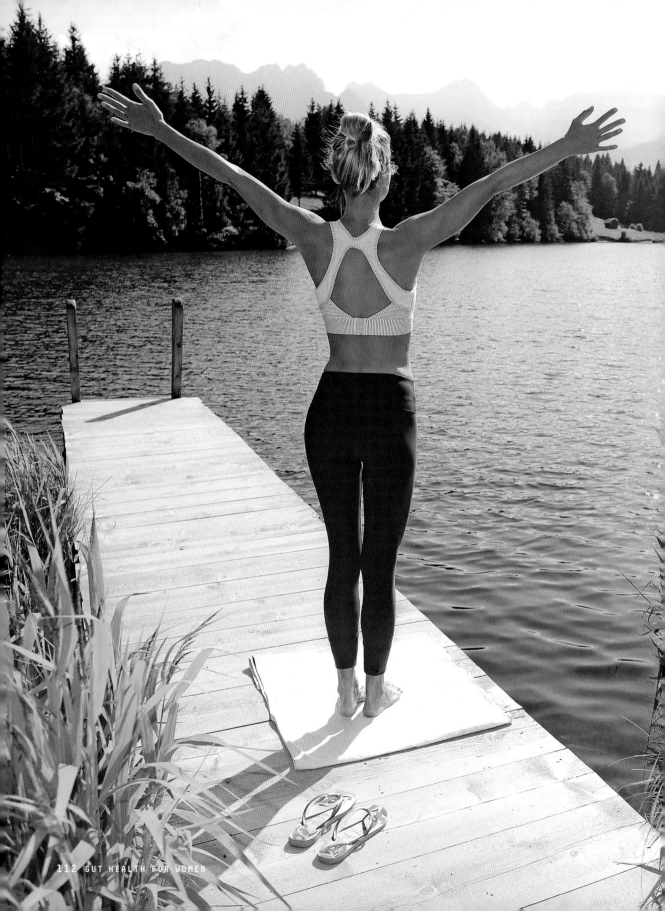

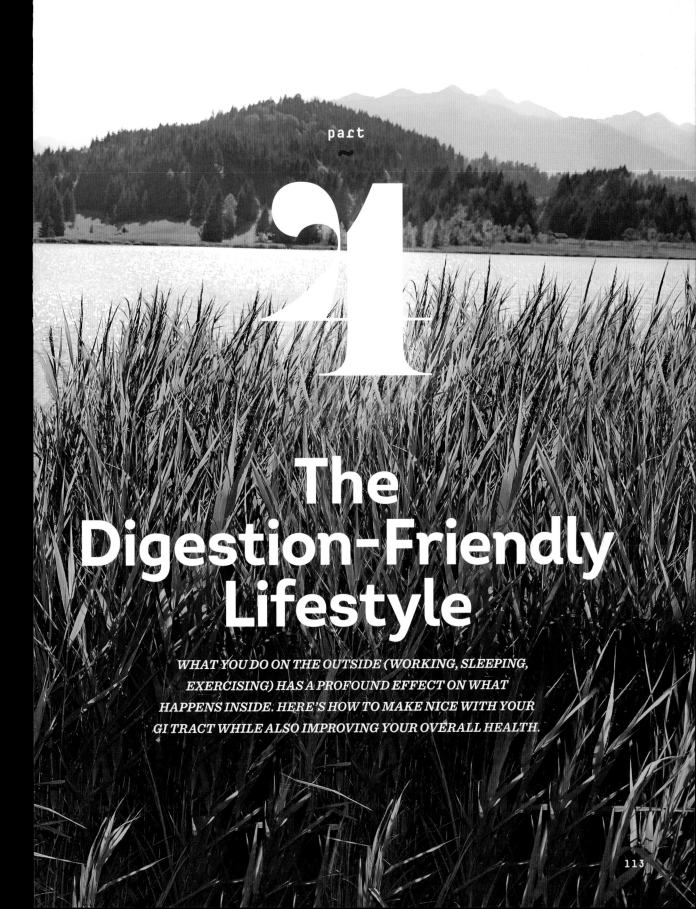

part

21

The Digestion-Friendly Lifestyle

WHAT YOU DO ON THE OUTSIDE (WORKING, SLEEPING, EXERCISING) HAS A PROFOUND EFFECT ON WHAT HAPPENS INSIDE. HERE'S HOW TO MAKE NICE WITH YOUR GI TRACT WHILE ALSO IMPROVING YOUR OVERALL HEALTH.

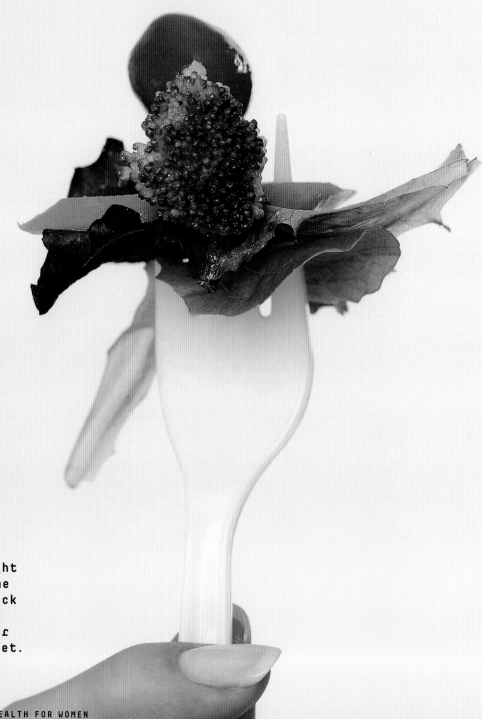

~

It might
be time
to stick
a fork
in your
old diet.

WEIGHT LOSS AND

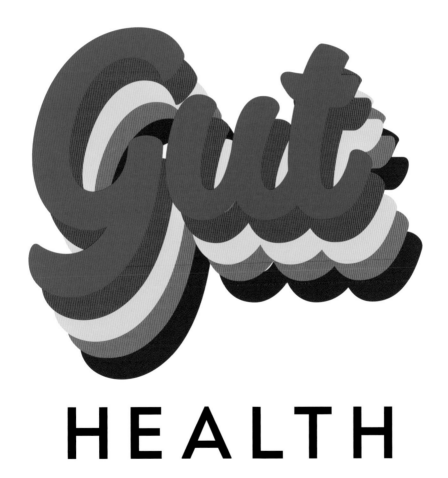

HEALTH

CALORIES ARE IMPORTANT, BUT YOUR MICROBIOME
MAY BE THWARTING YOUR EFFORTS TO PEEL OFF POUNDS.

you've been trying to lose weight and haven't been able to keep the number moving in the right direction, stop beating yourself up. A growing field of research suggests that, for some people, all the celery juice and keto diets in the world won't work, because their GI microbiome is messing with their weight. It may be that you need to improve your gut health to help shrink your waistline.

"It's new science," says Lauren Slayton, RD, founder of Foodtrainers and the author of *The Little Book of Thin*. "We know there is a connection between gut health and weight loss." Understanding exactly how this connection plays out is a work in progress —but in the meantime, there are things you can do to positively impact your gut health and possibly move the needle.

A Weighty Matter

In a study published in the *Proceedings of the National Academy of Sciences of the United States of America*, researchers divided sterile, germ-free mice into two groups. One received a microbiome transplant from obese mice, while the other received a transplant from lean mice. Although both groups ate the same diet, the ones who got the obese-mouse gut bacteria gained more weight.

"This was the first time we understood that microbes aren't just associated with

weight gain; they can actually *cause* weight gain," says Erica Sonnenburg, PhD, a research scientist at the Stanford University School of Medicine in the department of microbiology and immunology and co-author of *The Good Gut*. "It blew open the doors. This is a potent lever to control our metabolic rate."

Subsequent studies discovered that the microbiota in obese humans differs from the gut bacteria in lean humans. In a trial published in August 2018, Mayo Clinic scientists analyzed the gut microbes of 26 adults enrolled in an obesity-treatment program. According to their work, the bacteria Phascolarctobacterium was associated with weight-loss success, while the bacteria Dialister was associated with failure. And people with gut bacteria that more readily used carbohydrates for energy also tended to have a harder time losing.

While preliminary, the research suggests that, for some people, reducing caloric intake and being more active may not be enough to drop pounds. "There is something governing weight beyond willpower or what you decide to put into your mouth. It's like a control tower in the GI tract that drives what you crave, how quickly you get full, your appetite and more," Slayton says.

For one, the collection of microbes in the gut appears to dictate how many calories you extract from the foods you eat. "The microbes ferment complex carbohydrates, and then release waste products. Many of these are small chemicals that are absorbed into the bloodstream. We think that's one of the ways

Inflammation from "leaky gut" may thwart weight loss, too.

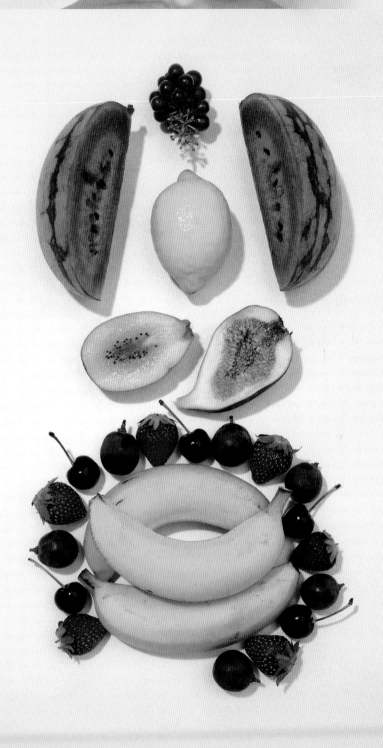

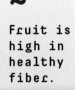

Fruit is
high in
healthy
fiber.

in which what you eat can influence your metabolism," Slayton explains. Additionally, these small chemicals may control appetite. "It's not a far stretch to think they could influence things like how hungry you feel," Sonnenburg says.

Gut health may also play a role in obesity via leaky gut syndrome. The gut is lined with mucus to keep too many toxins from entering the bloodstream. The lining stays strong, as long as the gut bacteria has food in the form of prebiotic fiber. But when you feed mice a diet that mimics the standard American diet—one that's high in simple sugars and animal-based fats, and low in dietary fiber—"the microbes consume the gut lining because there is no other food for them," Sonnenburg explains. "The layer gets thinner and the immune system senses that bacteria is close to the lining of the intestine, which sets off an inflammatory response. And obesity is an inflammatory disease."

Happy Bugs, Smaller Belly

For now, there isn't any specific "good gut diet." In fact, a study in the *International Journal of Obesity* in 2017 concluded what we already know: There is no single best diet. Rather, the scientists found that the ratio of Prevotella bacteria to Bacteroides bacteria in a person's colon determined how much body fat they lost on a certain diet.

But you can shift your eating to be more supportive of these beneficial microorganisms. The first step is understanding that "none of this will help if you're eating a crappy diet," Slayton stresses. "Sugary foods, refined carbs and artificial sweeteners are the worst." So try to limit or avoid baked goods, candy and white bread and pasta, as well as alcohol.

Then, feed your gut the foods that most experts recommend for overall health: plenty of fruit and vegetables; good fats; adequate

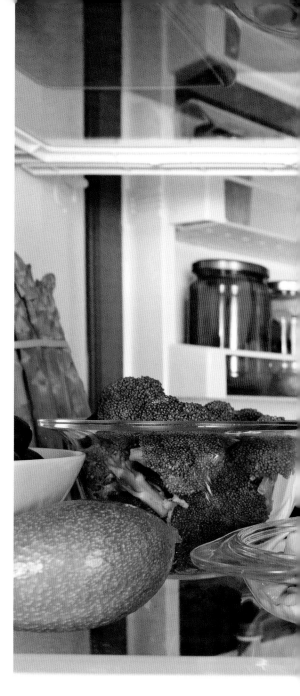

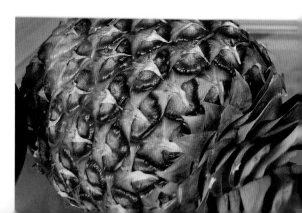

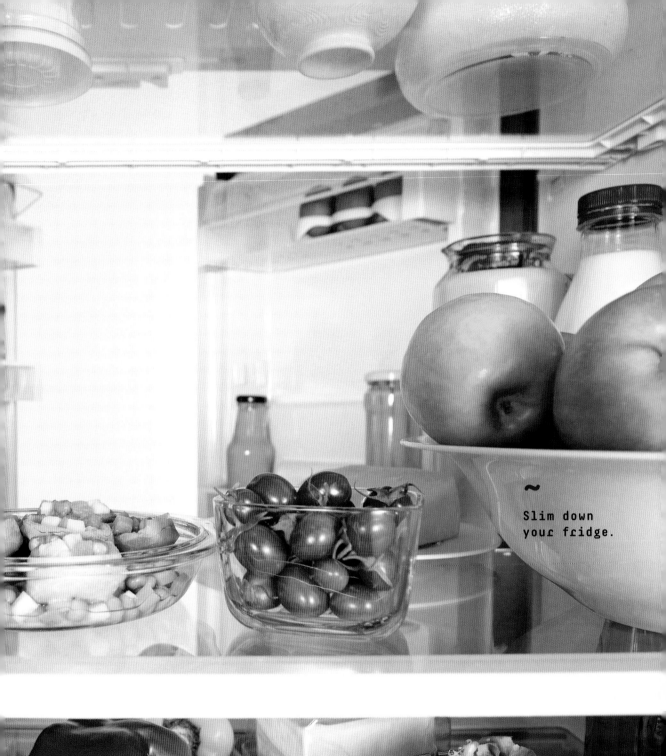

~
Slim down
your fridge.

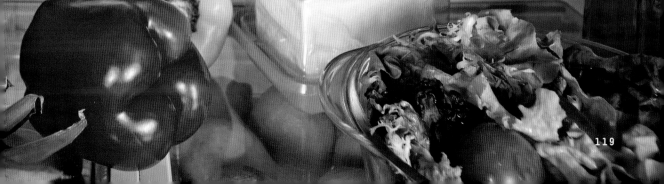

119

protein; and complex carbs. "That's baseline for having a healthy gut," Slayton says.

Sonnenburg agrees, adding that fiber from vegetables, fruit, nuts and legumes is key. "That's what really nourishes and promotes a microbiome that's highly diverse and is creating products that help regulate the immune system and metabolism," she says. And don't fall prey to thinking that carbohydrates are the devil because everyone you know is on the keto diet: Those low-carb plans may actually harm your gut. "With diets where you are not consuming carbs or are consuming them at very low levels, you are forcing your microbes to eat the mucus lining of the gut," Sonnenburg adds.

On top of a healthy balance of macronutrients, add in prebiotic foods (like onions, garlic, asparagus, plantains and sweet potatoes) for the healthy gut bacteria to feed on, as well as probiotic foods (like krauts, kimchi, miso, kombucha, kefir and yogurt) since this "good" gut bacteria brings benefits. But watch out that any kombucha, yogurt or kefir isn't loaded with added sugars. "If it has 20 grams of sugars, you're undoing the benefits that the bacteria provide," Sonnenburg says.

Lastly, you can't just have kefir at breakfast for a week and expect the scale to budge. "Things move quickly through your gastrointestinal tract and the real estate changes," Slayton says. In human trials with fecal transplants, people may lose weight for a short period of time, but then the pounds come right back on. "So if you want to get long-lasting benefits from these foods, you have to eat them on a regular basis. Otherwise, when you stop, the beneficial effects are going to disappear."

What about supplements? Although the research is mixed, Slayton considers them "an insurance policy." She recommends a probiotic that contains 10 to 12 different strains, and preferably Lactobacillus gasseri and Lactobacillus rhamnosus, which some studies say have weight-related benefits.

In one study published in the *British Journal of Nutrition*, adults consumed 200 grams of fermented milk containing Lactobacillus gasseri every day for 12 weeks. At the end of the trial, some had lost 8.5 percent of their belly fat. And in a review of 21 studies published in *Genes* in 2018, the use of probiotics significantly reduced BMI, weight and fat mass compared to a placebo. When researchers compared single-species probiotics, Lactobacillus probiotics showed the greatest reductions in body weight and fat mass.

Taking *prebiotics* also significantly reduced body weight compared to taking a placebo, which the study authors say may be due to their ability to reduce appetite and improve lipid metabolism.

Just keep in mind that supplements will only help with weight loss if you're doing other things correctly, Slayton says. You cannot out-supplement an unhealthy diet.

Prebiotics can help boost fat metabolism and insulin sensitivity.

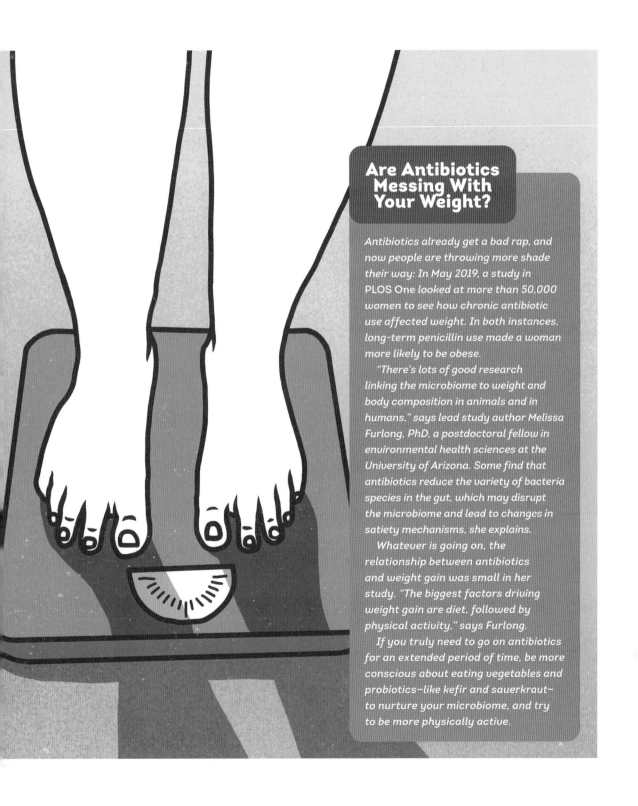

Are Antibiotics Messing With Your Weight?

Antibiotics already get a bad rap, and now people are throwing more shade their way: In May 2019, a study in PLOS One looked at more than 50,000 women to see how chronic antibiotic use affected weight. In both instances, long-term penicillin use made a woman more likely to be obese.

"There's lots of good research linking the microbiome to weight and body composition in animals and in humans," says lead study author Melissa Furlong, PhD, a postdoctoral fellow in environmental health sciences at the University of Arizona. Some find that antibiotics reduce the variety of bacteria species in the gut, which may disrupt the microbiome and lead to changes in satiety mechanisms, she explains.

Whatever is going on, the relationship between antibiotics and weight gain was small in her study. "The biggest factors driving weight gain are diet, followed by physical activity," says Furlong.

If you truly need to go on antibiotics for an extended period of time, be more conscious about eating vegetables and probiotics—like kefir and sauerkraut— to nurture your microbiome, and try to be more physically active.

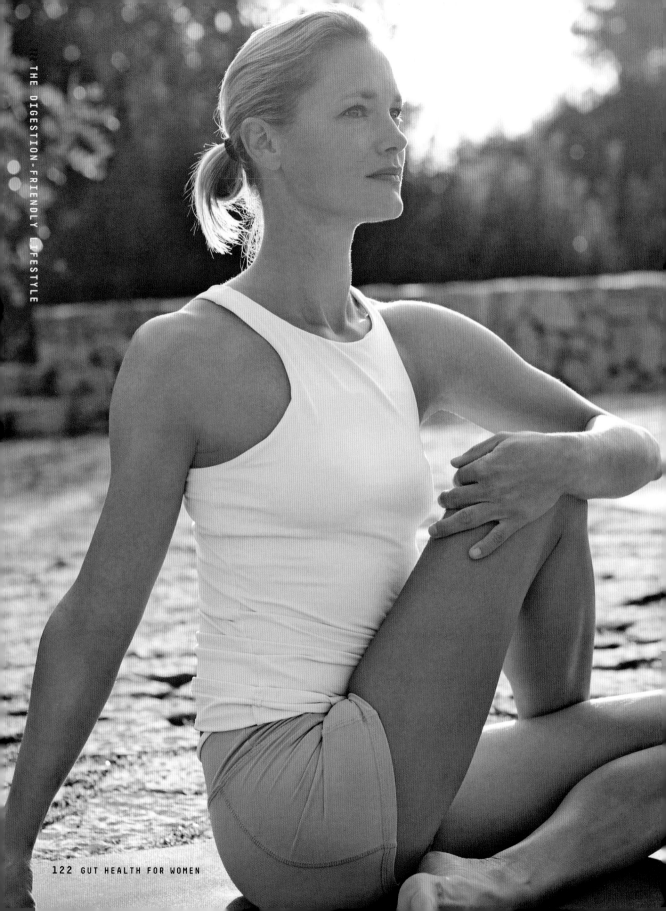

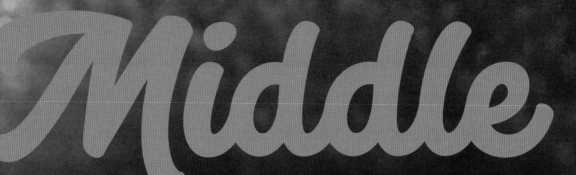

Middle
MANAGEMENT

*NEW RESEARCH IS SHOWING
REGULAR EXERCISE DOES MORE
FOR YOUR BODY THAN BOOST
HEART HEALTH AND BURN CALORIES.*

You're probably starting to understand that the healthier your lifestyle is—a good diet high in fiber, adequate sleep, low levels of stress—the happier and more diverse the organisms that live in your digestive tract will be. The same holds true for that other element of a good-for-you way of life: exercise. Sure, being active helps your heart and circulatory system work better; lowers your risk of a multitude of diseases; keeps your stress levels low and your mental health on an even keel—but it also seems to have a direct impact on those trillions of bugs toiling away in your colon. The more active you are, the better the odds of having a thriving microbiome.

The interplay between these tiny bugs and the rest of the body is complex and multifaceted, especially when it comes to working out. The bacteria—via the byproducts of their daily smorgasbord—are what fuel your body during exercise.

According to a review published in *Frontiers in Physiology*, "The genetic information encoded in all the microorganisms acquired from the environment (collectively known as the microbiome) also regulates mitochondrial functions by modifying energy production, ROS [reactive oxygen species] production, inflammatory responses and transcription factors involved in mitochondrial biogenesis [coding for more energy pumps in the cells]." That's jargon for: The microbiome gives you serious oomph to get through your workouts!

But it's a two-way street. The mitochondria, the energy-fuel pumps within each cell in the human body, also impact the gut by aiding the immune response and helping maintain the intestinal barrier. The more endurance exercise you do, the more mitochondria are created to fuel the muscles. Exercise may also alter the gut microbiota by affecting the amount of body fat. Various studies have shown that excess body fat can decrease microbial diversity, potentially impacting gut health.

"You can't compartmentalize the body," says Lauryn Nyhoff, metabolic specialist and nutrition coach at Life Time fitness center in Omaha, Nebraska. "What you do in one aspect will affect another. The gut and exercise are related through the nervous system. The gut has its own nervous system and tends to respond very sensitively to different nutritional and exercise interventions. Exercise, especially intense workouts, puts a stress on the body, which teaches the body to be resilient and handle more stress. The gut responds to that."

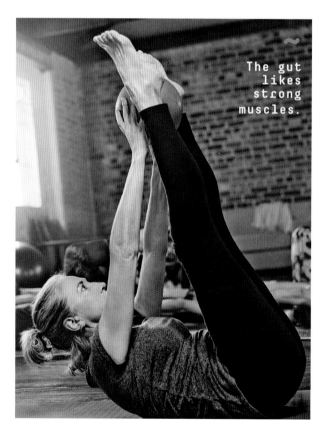

The gut likes strong muscles.

Aerobics for Your Colon

Besides its relationship with the residents of your GI tract, exercise is also good medicine for general digestive complaints, such as nausea, bloating and constipation. Working out helps stimulate movement through the GI tract and improves blood flow to the entire body, including the gut. A recent review found that exercise significantly improved constipation symptoms. Even yoga, which involves twisting movements as well as mindfulness training that can help reduce stress, can stimulate your GI tract to move things along.

Get Fit Faster

The American College of Sports Medicine recommends accumulating at least 30 minutes of moderate aerobic exercise daily for overall health. If you do more intense exercise, you only need to accumulate 75 minutes a week (in addition to strength and flexibility exercises). To improve cardiovascular fitness, though, you need to regularly challenge your system.

When it comes to getting fit, it's all a matter of intensity, says Nyhoff. Different intensities prompt different physiological responses. "At Life Time, we have three different categories for programs that we've labeled 'sustain,' 'gain' and 'pain,' based on the intensity level. You should incorporate all three in your workout program to improve fitness." (Don't let that "pain" part put you off; those types of workouts are usually super-short since they're so intense.) Here's how it works:

SUSTAIN (two or more days a week)

This is a moderate-intensity, aerobic workout that builds endurance. It trains your body to get really efficient at using fat for fuel. Pick an intensity you can maintain for 30 to 40 minutes, one where you're able to hold a conversation but not sing. Run, bike, walk or use the elliptical or rower; just choose an activity you enjoy.

GAIN (once a week)

This is where intervals—alternating bursts of higher-intensity activity with lower-intensity recovery—come in. Go hard for two or three minutes and rest for one minute (or make your work and rest periods equal). You're at a level where you can't maintain a conversation, but you can say a few words at a time. Do this kind of workout on a cardio machine, or with body-weight exercises.

PAIN (once a week)

These intervals are challenging but over fast. Try going as hard as you can for 30 seconds, then resting for a minute (the less you rest, the more intense it becomes). You'll probably only be able to say one word while doing these but you won't want to talk. Do these intervals on a cardio machine and add resistance, speed or both.

Get It Done at Home

Don't belong to a gym? Never underestimate the power of your own body to help you work up a sweat. Besides walking, running, skating, rowing or biking outside, there are plenty of online programs that can help you get fit fast.

KIRA STOKES FIT APP

New York celebrity trainer Stokes (she works with Ashley Graham and Norah O'Donnell, among others) is the queen of creative body-weight and minimal-equipment moves. You'll get everything from quickie workouts (six-minute toning blocks) to an hourlong total body cardio and strength bonanza. ($15 per month after a seven-day free intro)

GLO (formerly YogaGlo)

This online yoga portal (also available via app) offers a variety of classes with top yogis, including Sara Clark, Kathryn Budig, Amy Ippoliti and Richard Freeman. Want something more intense? Opt for yoga conditioning. Need to chill? You'll find yoga nidra and yin yoga. Search based on level, focus, teacher, length and more. ($18 per month after a 15-day free trial)

DAILY BURN

If you like a ton of variety in your workouts, dailyburn.com (available via app) is the place. You can enjoy on-demand classes for all levels, including yoga, strength training, barre, dance, Pilates and boxing. Celebrity trainers make cameo appearances to help motivate you to work harder than you did last time. ($15 per month after a 30-day free trial)

The Stress-GI

Dis

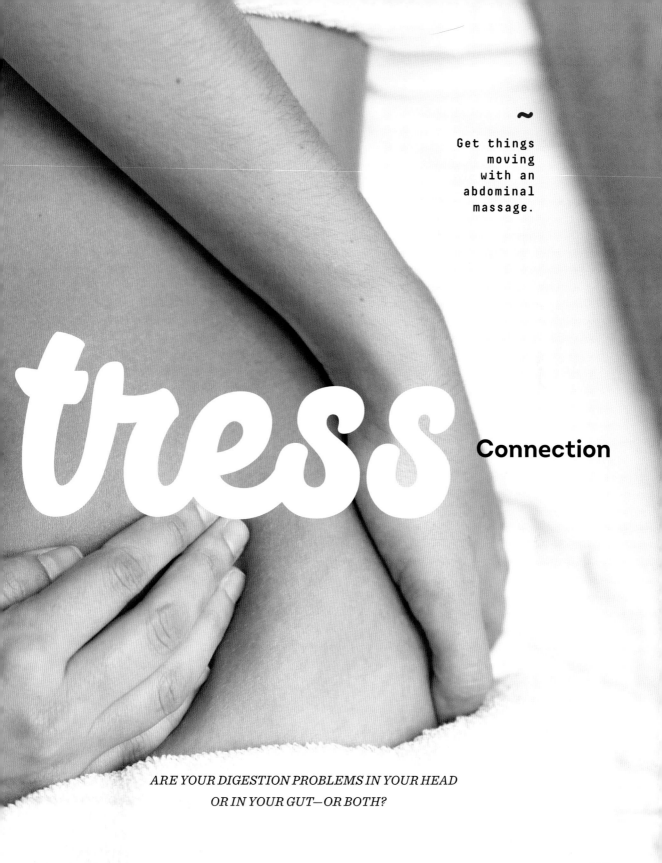

~

Get things
moving
with an
abdominal
massage.

tress **Connection**

ARE YOUR DIGESTION PROBLEMS IN YOUR HEAD

OR IN YOUR GUT—OR BOTH?

You have noticed your stomach rumbling more, and you're bloated, but you chalk it up to the crazy deadline you've been racing to meet at work. Sure, stress can wreak havoc on your gastrointestinal system—from triggering reflux to slowing down or speeding up your bowel movements—but the relationship is more complicated, and it's rooted in that huge colony of microorganisms teeming in your colon.

"Stress hormones are produced in the adrenal glands. The hypothalamic-pituitary-adrenal (HPA) axis [the conduit for hormone communication between the brain and the adrenals] develops correctly when there's good gut health from birth, especially a vaginal birth," says Laura Rokosz, PhD, founder of EgglRock Nutrition in Union, New Jersey. "That's why it's so important, no matter how you give birth, to do everything you can to foster the growth of good bacteria. That will drive the development of that HPA axis."

That connection really comes into play as an adult. Research has shown that stress can lead to gut dysbiosis, an alteration in the normal homeostasis of the bacteria. And that can trigger digestive issues that cause emotional and mental stress.

It doesn't matter whether you're experiencing gas, bloating, reflux, constipation, abdominal pain or diarrhea; they're all sensitive to stress, says gut specialist Laurie Keefer, PhD, a clinical psychologist at NYC's Mount Sinai School of Medicine's division of gastroenterology. "If I think broadly about GI issues, all of them are stress-sensitive disorders," she says. Conditions like IBS are much more closely tied to stress, while Crohn's and ulcerative colitis, which have an underlying organic cause, are less controlled by it, although they're still susceptible. "IBS is a motility and brain-gut dysregulation problem by definition," Keefer explains. "In that condition, stress is directly acting on it; it's largely the cause. If you have a digestive disease, you have to be more proactive in managing your stress than other people do."

The vagus nerve facilitates communication between the gut and brain, and it's the pathway to turning down the stress. "The vagus nerve runs from the brain to the gut and they're in constant communication. It's also very sensitive to disruption," says Keefer. "We're really seeing from the data that the relationship between gut and brain is bidirectional. People think, 'I wouldn't have stress if I didn't have these [GI] symptoms. The symptoms are what's stressing me out.' No, your gut issues are being amplified at the brain level because of a fear of symptoms or catastrophizing of symptoms. Then the brain perceives the threat and activates the sympathetic nervous system."

"I really believe that stress is almost more important than food when it comes to impacting your gut health," says Carley Smith, NTP, creator of the Fairy Gutmother blog, who specializes in working with clients who have gut issues. "I see it firsthand with clients and the research that I've been able to help with. I see it reflected in the microbiome."

A study at Brigham Young University in Provo, Utah, found that female mice who were

TIP
A simple mantra like "om" can help you focus while meditating.

"Stress is almost more important than food for gut health."

Nutrition therapist Carley Smith

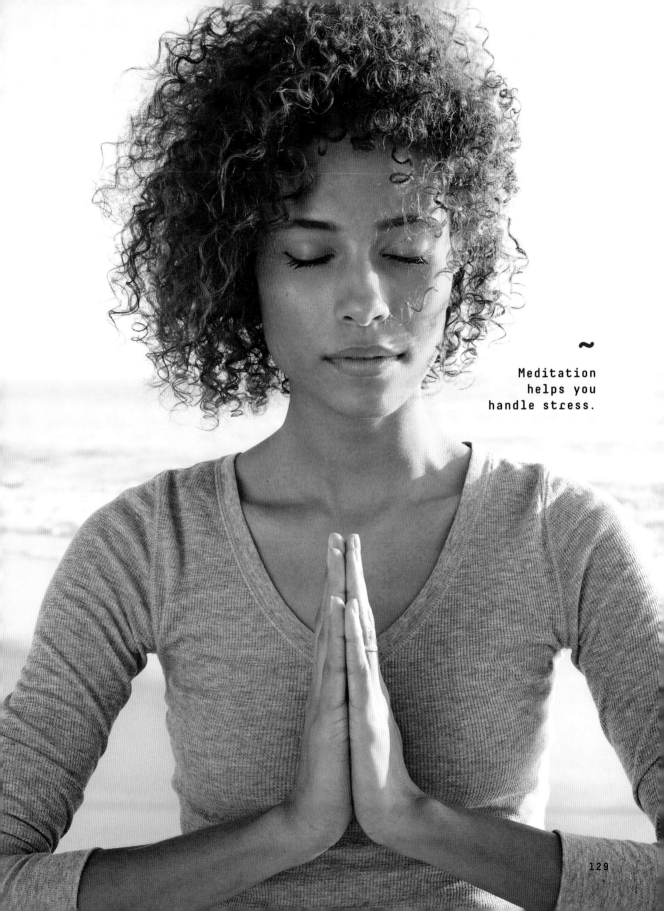

~
Meditation
helps you
handle stress.

129

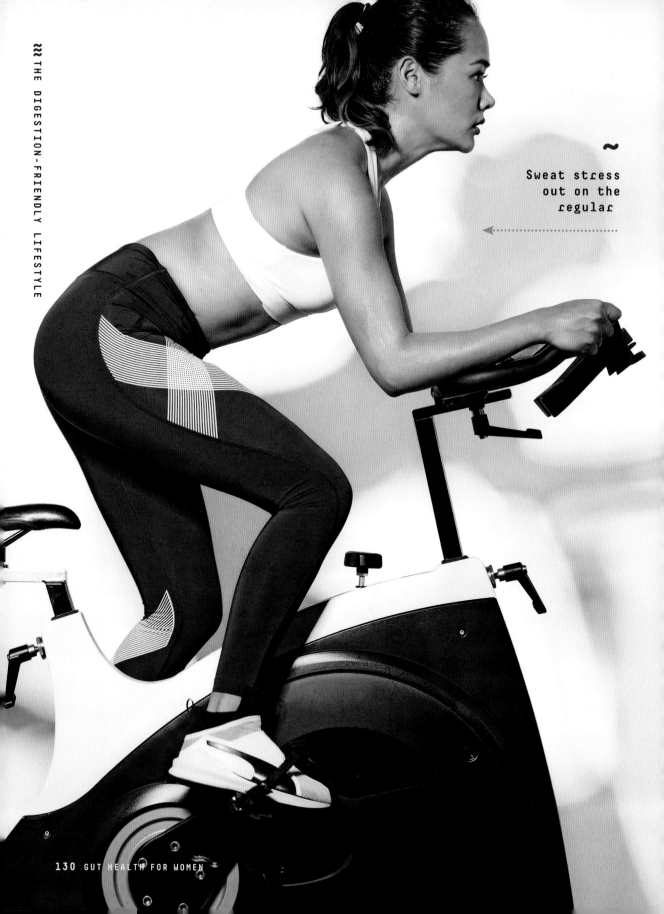

~

Sweat stress out on the regular

put under stress experienced unhealthy changes in their gut microbiota that were comparable to what happens when you eat a high-fat diet. (Male mice didn't see the same effect; researchers speculate gut-bacteria changes may be to blame for the higher rates of depression and anxiety in women.) "I'll see people who have a really healthy diet but high stress levels, and then clients with OK diets and moderate to mild stress," says Smith. "When I send in a sample to sequence the microbiome, more times than not, the high-stress/good-diet group's guts are not well-diversified. They have very few species of anti-inflammatory bacteria and there's an increase in pathogenic bacteria like E. coli. Stress absolutely wreaks havoc on the gut."

Smith's experience shows that having a healthy gut is all about lifestyle. "It's diet combined with managing stress, taking time out for self-care, getting outside and exercising. People are so overstimulated and it's really showing in the gut."

If you need to start reducing your stress levels yesterday, give the following a try.

Sit and Meditate

Taking time to get quiet and bring your attention to your breath or a mantra isn't necessarily calming in and of itself. In fact, it can feel like hard work just sitting still. Then, as one thought after another intrudes on your efforts, you have to keep tugging your focus back to your breath. But in that hard work, you'll learn the skills that will help you when you are feeling stressed or your thoughts start to spiral. If you're interested in learning how to meditate, start with just a few minutes each day, maybe right after waking or before your first cup of coffee, and build from there.

Get Bendy

There are many types of yoga, and each one emphasizes mindfulness and a focus on the body and breath. Active types (hatha, vinyasa, Ashtanga and hot yoga) tackle stress in two ways: The exercise aspect itself is cathartic, and the mindfulness part helps pull the brain away from your anxiety-provoking thoughts. If you just need to be chill, look for a yin yoga class that emphasizes held stretches and an opportunity to train the sympathetic nervous system to step down. Yoga nidra classes are even more relaxing and involve very little movement.

Talk It Out

Working with a licensed therapist or counselor can provide new insight into what exactly is triggering the stress you feel—and give you tools to tackle it. Cognitive behavioral therapy (CBT) is an increasingly common technique that really puts the patient in the driver's seat. "It's a short-term, collaborative skills–based therapy focused on improving symptom management," says Keefer, who uses it with her GI patients. "I'm giving them real-life skills to deal with their issues. For pretty much any GI patient, I always give them a way to control their nervous system response, such as a deep breathing technique, hypnosis, mindfulness or progressive muscle relaxation."

77% of people regularly show physical symptoms of stress.

Source: American Institute of Stress

Head for Green

Many studies have looked at the benefits of getting out in nature, whether it's in an urban park or a secluded forest (the farther away from the city, the better). One 2018 study published in the journal *Evidence-Based Complementary and Alternative Medicine* found that walking outdoors in a city and in a bamboo forest both decreased blood pressure and brain activity, but only the latter significantly reduced anxiety and improved mood. A new trend called forest bathing, or *shinrin-yoku*, involves immersing yourself in a forest (or whatever green space you can find) and noticing your surroundings by engaging all your senses. But don't overthink it: A good hike or trail run will also help get the job done.

Work Up a Sweat

Physical activity—whether it's tennis, dance class, walking the dog or a boxing lesson—helps turn down the volume on stress by switching the nervous system from fight-or-flight to rest-and-recover. Despite the fact that exercise is a physical stressor (that boxing class more so than walking the dog), the end effect is it kicks on the parasympathetic, stress-busting response while also releasing feel-good endorphins in the brain. The American College of Sports Medicine recommends getting at least 30 minutes of moderate exercise (less if you're doing vigorous workouts) on most days of the week and two or three strength-training sessions weekly.

Soothe From the Inside

While you may want to reach for that box of mac and cheese when you're feeling stressed, you're better off plating up some roasted veggies. Studies have linked oxidative stress—the kind caused by damaging free radicals—to anxiety, and the best foods we have to fight it are plants that are high in antioxidants. Think: leafy greens, berries (especially blueberries), green tea, coffee and legumes. Besides fighting the little chemical marauders, these foods are also high in fiber, so they help promote good gut health. That means your colon is less likely to send up the red flag via the vagus nerve. Since stress can also trigger inflammation, add in some seafood (such as salmon) and flaxseed for anti-inflammatory, brain-boosting omega-3s. Belly's happy, brain's happy, you're happy.

A Better Type of Massage?

A relaxing rubdown on a warm table while you're serenaded by spa music: That's the ideal stress reliever for many people. But there's a massage that tackles the gut in particular, releasing tension—and emotions—you may not have known were there.

"So many people hold their stress and other emotions in their abdomen, and that can restrict movement through the GI tract, leading to bloating, reflux, pain and more. Abdominal massage helps release tension, as well as physical adhesions, which promotes movement," says Alex Jackson, LMT, owner of Centered Spirit Cultural and Holistic Center in Kansas City, Missouri. Studies have shown it can increase the number and weight of bowel movements, in addition to reducing straining.

If you go, expect firm pressure, from the sternum to your pubic bone and from side to side.

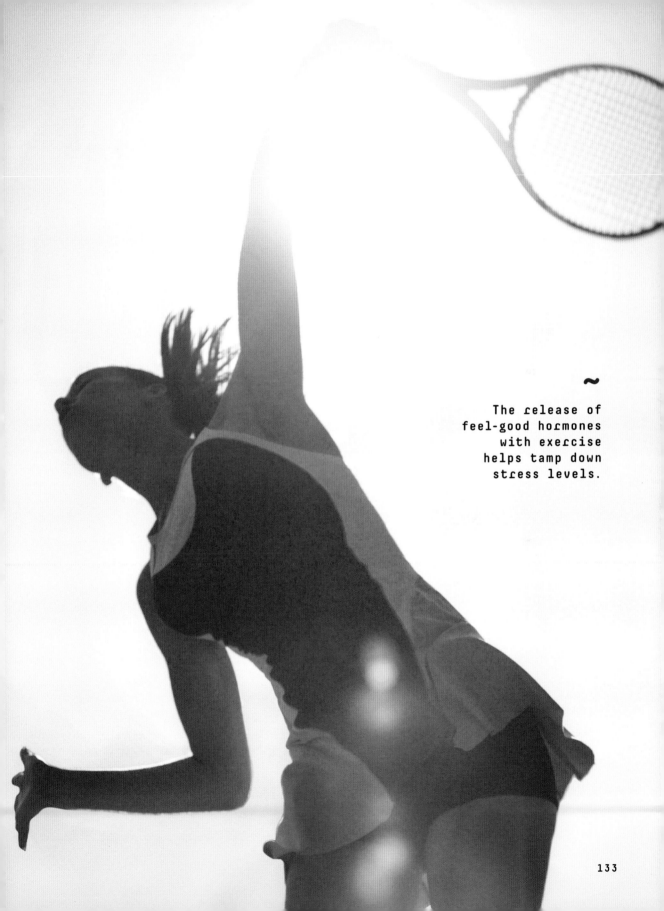

The release of
feel-good hormones
with exercise
helps tamp down
stress levels.

~

Put some
glow into
your diet.

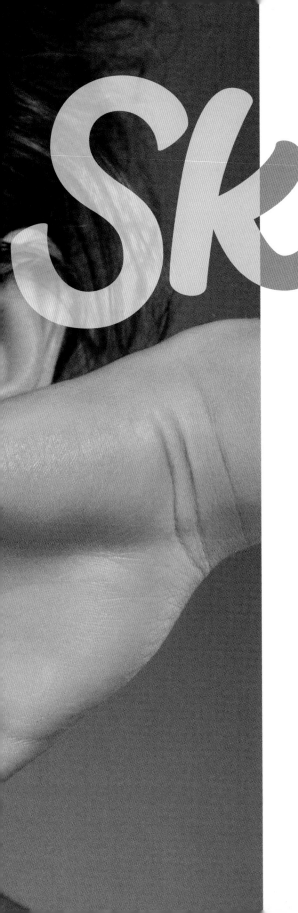

Skin

SECRETS

*GETTING BEAUTIFUL
ON THE OUTSIDE IS AN INSIDE JOB.*

P erhaps the old adage "you are what you eat" should be "you look like what you eat." Maybe you've noticed how when you snack on foods high in sugar, such as candy bars and cookies, you tend to break out. Or how your vegan sister-in-law seems to have the most glowing, dewy skin you've ever seen in real life. "We used to think about the gut microbiome in isolation from the rest of the body. Now we know it plays an important role in other organ systems, such as the immune system, cardiovascular system—and even the skin," says Shilpi Khetarpal, MD, a dermatologist at the Cleveland Clinic in Ohio. "When the normal balance of bacteria, viruses, fungi and protozoa in the gut is off [aka dysbiosis], it can affect the skin."

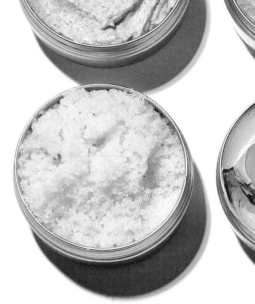

Researchers continue to learn more about how gut health is connected to specific skin conditions such as acne, psoriasis, eczema and rosacea. Their insights will help lead to better treatments, but why wait for science?

Your Window Into the Gut

The exact connection between the gut and skin is unclear, but the immune system seems to play a role. The good bacteria in the gut microbiome produce beneficial molecules, including short-chain fatty acids and digestive enzymes. These compounds improve immunity and help trigger anti-inflammatory responses. But other harmful gut microbes and metabolites promote inflammation. And many skin conditions, including eczema, psoriasis and rosacea, are inflammatory conditions.

Additionally, when you don't eat enough prebiotics from fibrous foods to feed the good bacteria in the gut, unhealthy bacteria can take over. "As the bad bugs begin to outnumber the good bugs, the gut lining becomes compromised," explains Whitney Bowe, MD, a New York–based dermatologist and co-author of *The Beauty of Dirty Skin*. Known as leaky gut, this can allow harmful bacteria to enter the bloodstream, causing inflammation throughout the body, including the skin.

Your outer layer claims its own microbiome too, which forms a barrier to help keep pathogens out and prevent infection. But when this microbiome is out of balance, the barrier is less resilient. "It's no longer preventing allergens and irritants from entering the epidermis [outer layer of skin], and it's unable to adequately trap moisture in the skin to keep it healthy and hydrated," Bowe says. In a 2001 study of 114 people with acne, more than half had an impaired intestinal microbiota.

Exercise and sleep also play a role in good skin.

The bacteria Cutibacterium acnes has also been linked to acne for more than a century. C. acnes in the skin microbiota appears to promote the production of sebum, the formation of pimples, and inflammation.

The third player here is the brain. "The gut, brain and skin all communicate with each other," Khetarpal explains. Compounds produced in the gut also send signals to the brain. "These signals can improve our mood and stress level, and when you have stress, it can affect your skin," says Mahmoud A. Ghannoum, PhD, director of the Center for Medical Mycology and Integrated Microbiome Core at Case Western Reserve University in

TIP
Go fragrance-free to avoid inflammation triggers.

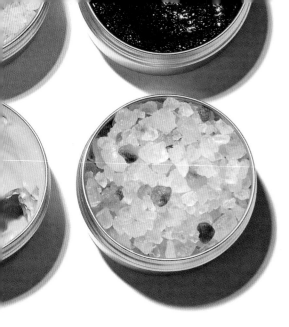

Ohio. For example, studies show stress can trigger acne, psoriasis and atopic dermatitis.

It's not just stress. Patients with psoriasis also have an imbalance in gut bacteria and fungi. In fact, 7 to 11 percent of people with inflammatory bowel disease are also diagnosed with psoriasis, according to a 2018 study. And it appears that rosacea may be connected to small intestinal bacterial overgrowth (SIBO). In two studies, 46 percent of patients with rosacea had this condition, compared with just 5 to 10 percent of healthy people.

Research has also found that people who have eczema don't only have different bacteria in their gut compared to those without eczema; they also sometimes have an inflamed gut and an altered skin microbiome in affected areas.

A Plan for Radiant Skin

"In order to have clear, healthy skin, you have to first heal your gut. The fastest way to do this is to limit the foods that cause inflammation," Bowe says. Avoid processed foods, and if you consume dairy, stick with cheese and yogurt with live cultures and minimal added sugars.

Cutting back on processed foods will also help you reduce your intake of added sugars. "Refined carbohydrates and sugars have been scientifically linked to acne and premature

aging, among other serious health issues," Bowe says. Then "add anti-inflammatory, fiber-filled, low-glycemic index, nutrient-rich options," Bowe recommends. When you want carbs, reach for minimally processed ones, like steel-cut oats, quinoa, sweet potatoes or wild rice. And don't forget about food sources of probiotics, such as miso or kefir.

A probiotic supplement can also help. "Several strains of Lactobacillus have anti-inflammatory properties that help reduce the risk of skin disorders," Bowe says. "They have also been shown to improve the strength of the skin barrier, and they can potentially protect skin from the damaging effects of UV rays."

Feed Your Face

This homemade **Probiotic Power Mask** recipe from New York City–based dermatologist Whitney Bowe, MD, is great for all skin types: "Jojoba is naturally antibacterial, hypoallergenic, anti-inflammatory, able to relieve pain, and it penetrates the skin deeply to really nourish. Honey is antibacterial and anti-inflammatory, and the probiotics pack an added punch of healing goodness," she explains. (Spot-test the recipe on your neck or behind an ear to be certain that none of the ingredients irritates your skin.)

1 teaspoon jojoba oil
1 teaspoon raw organic honey
2–3 probiotics capsules (look for those with multiple strains, including Lactobacillus)

INSTRUCTIONS:
In a small bowl, combine oil, honey and probiotics (open capsules and sprinkle in contents) and mix well. Apply to clean skin, let sit for 15 to 20 minutes, then rinse with warm water and a soft washcloth. Pat skin dry.

SNOOZE YOUR WAY TO A

Happy Belly

THERE'S A SURPRISING LINK BETWEEN YOUR NIGHTLY Z'S AND YOUR DIGESTION.

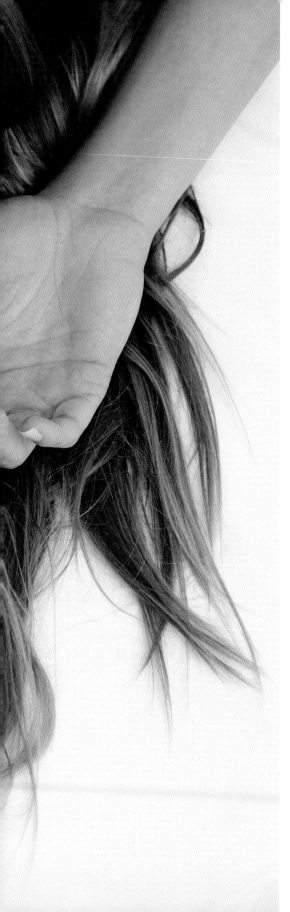

t's 3 a.m. and you're lying
awake in bed again, listening to
your stomach gurgle and groan.
You toss and turn, trying to find
a position that quiets the noises
or eases the discomfort. Is it something
you ate? Or could the real culprit be the
less than six hours of sleep you've been
running on for the past month?*

There are many potential causes of digestive
issues like acid reflux, gas, bloating, diarrhea,
constipation and abdominal pain, from allergic
and autoimmune reactions to stress and diet.
But more recent research suggests that sleep
(both quality and quantity) holds more sway
over digestive health—and the tiny bugs that
make it tick—than we realized.

Meet Your Biological Middle Man

"The gut microbiome refers to a network
of microorganisms (mostly bacteria) that
reside inside the gastrointestinal tract, aid
digestion and influence a range of biological
and neurochemical processes throughout
the body and brain," says Scott Anderson,
co-author of *The Psychobiotic Revolution*.
Some of the microorganisms that make up
the microbiome are present in your belly from
birth. Others are introduced into the gut via
the environments you spend time in. Think:
the water you drink, the air you breathe and
the soil your food comes from. The gut flora
have a separate (and more complex) genomic
structure than our own human cells do, and
their function and diversity can be altered by
diet, exercise and sleep habits.

Gut flora play a role in the concentration of acid within the intestines, the extraction of nutrients from food, the elimination of waste and the consistency of your stool—just for starters. They also heavily influence the production of key hormones and neurotransmitters involved in the sleep-wake cycle. Lactobacillus rhamnosus lives naturally in the gut, and it's also found in sauerkraut, kimchi and some yogurts. This probiotic has gained fame in the scientific community for reducing diarrhea, preventing some forms of dermatitis and protecting against UTIs. It has also been shown to affect the expression of gamma-Aminobutyric acid (GABA), a neurochemical that helps you relax and fall asleep by inhibiting excitatory signaling in the brain. "Various bacteria in the gut also play a role in producing the sleep-inducing hormone melatonin," says Lisa Richards, a certified nutritionist and co-author of *The Ultimate Candida Diet.* "Research also suggests that bacteria within the gut help facilitate the production of the mood-modulating neurotransmitter serotonin, which is a chemical precursor to melatonin."

Where Things Go Wrong

"The concentration of good bacteria teeming in the gut—and the quality of your digestive health—can be disrupted by poor sleep. But a dip in the abundance of good bacteria caused by other factors—such as stress, diet, exposure to environmental toxins (like cigarette smoke) and antibiotic use—can also cause or worsen sleep issues," says Richards. This creates a vicious cycle where poor sleep can cause or exacerbate imbalances in gut bacteria, and imbalances in gut bacteria or digestive issues can lead to poor sleep.

Insufficient snoozing has been shown to reduce the concentration of beneficial bacteria in the gut, clearing more space for pathogen bacteria (such as E. coli and salmonella) and yeast, which can cause infection and disease. Shift workers, who experience brief, interrupted sleep patterns, are more likely to have an imbalance between beneficial and harmful bacteria in their guts. This has been shown to weaken their immune systems, leaving them more vulnerable to everything from colds to different types of cancers and cardiovascular disease.

But it doesn't take a career as a shift worker to throw your system out of whack. A 2016 study found that just two nights of sleep deprivation (less than five hours) led to a decrease in beneficial gut bacteria among healthy young men with otherwise regular sleep patterns. Another consequence of brief sleep deprivation? Metabolic changes linked to obesity and diabetes, like greater insulin resistance.

"Just as the rest of your body requires downtime to recharge and replenish, so too does the microbiome," says registered dietitian Diane Welland, author of *The Complete Idiot's Guide to Eating Clean.* Inadequate sleep deprives the microbiome of the chance to flush out harmful bacteria and recalibrate its balance of beneficial bacteria, leading to that buildup of bad bugs that can trigger or exacerbate digestive issues like bowel irregularity and IBS—not to mention leaving you susceptible to foodborne illnesses.

An abundance of harmful bacteria in the digestive tract can also produce neurotoxins like ammonia that trigger the vagus nerve to increase stress hormones or alter the production of neurochemicals involved in sleep-wake cycles, says Anderson.

Increased stress itself worsens digestive issues, thanks to the effect of stress hormones on the digestive tract, and ratchets up inflammation, which increases vulnerability to digestive health issues.

STOP THE CYCLE

LIMIT FRIED AND PROCESSED FOODS These have been found to disrupt the balance of beneficial bacteria in the colons.

EAT FOODS THAT KEEP THE BUGS HAPPY "Bone broth contains an amino acid called glutamine that can reduce intestinal inflammation caused by gut dysbiosis, an imbalance between good and bad bacteria, with the bad outweighing the good," Richards explains. Kefir, which contains a symbiotic collection of bacteria and yeast, is also easy on your digestive system and is rich in nutrients, as is fermented or probiotic yogurt.

GET MOVING Exercise can favorably alter intestinal flora, improve sleep quality, and help resolve constipation, bloating, gas and other IBS symptoms. Just a brisk 30-minute walk on most days, plus two or three weightlifting sessions per week, can make a difference. If a full half-hour seems out of the question, try doing three bouts of 10 minutes throughout the day. Research suggests this still confers benefits.

Foods That Make You Go "ZZZZZ"

Studies have shown there are some specific foods that can help you fall asleep faster and get more quality rest. Consider adding these to your grocery list.

KIWI *Eating two kiwi fruits within an hour of bedtime for one month was found to significantly increase the quality and length of sleep in adults with sleep disorders in a 2011 study. (The fuzzy fruits are a good source of fiber and are also helpful for constipation and other IBS symptoms.)*

CHAMOMILE TEA *This herb has been shown to help promote sleep in many studies. It may be because the chemicals in chamomile contain a flavonoid compound called apigenin, which stimulates neurons in the brain that are involved in sedation. (Apigenin is a polyphenol; they are being studied for their potentially positive benefit on gut bugs.)*

WALNUTS *If you're hankering for some crunch, consider throwing back a handful of walnuts with dinner or as a late-night snack. Thanks to their high concentration of melatonin, walnuts have been found to promote sleep. (One ounce contains almost 2 grams of fiber, too.)*

FATTY FISH *Eating omega-3-rich fish, like salmon, may improve sleep quality and duration. A 2014 study published in the Journal of Clinical Sleep Medicine found that men who consumed salmon three times per week reported better sleep than those who consumed beef, chicken or pork alone. A 2017 study of children in China found a strong positive correlation between how much fish children consumed and how well they slept.*

TART CHERRY JUICE *Drinking one cup of tart cherry juice with breakfast and dinner for two weeks significantly reduced insomnia symptoms among older adults in a 2010 study at Rochester University. Another study, published in the European Journal of Nutrition, found that noninsomniac adults saw improvements in their sleep quality after the same intervention. Researchers point to the high melatonin concentration of tart cherries.*

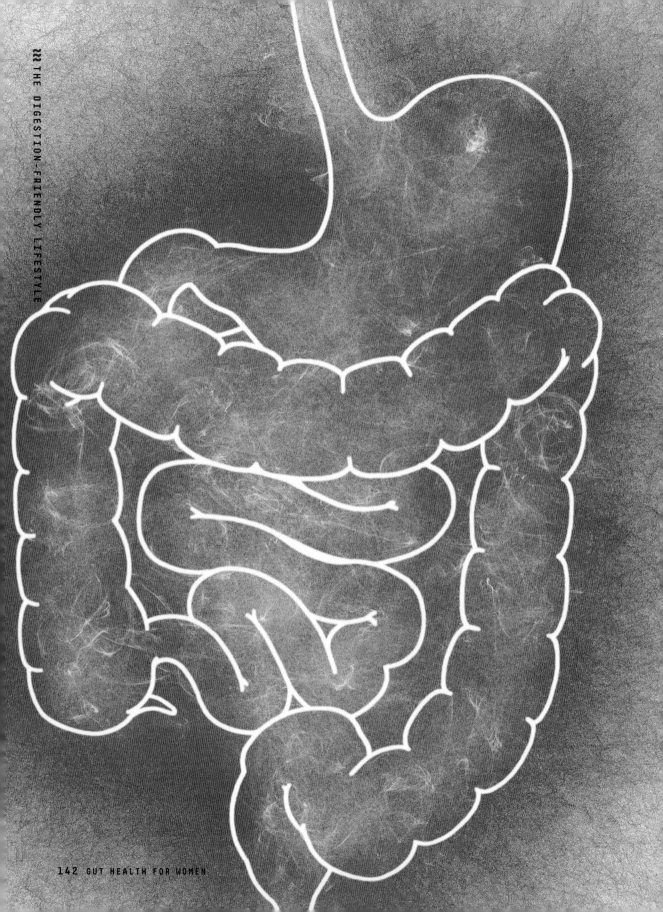

I FIXED MY

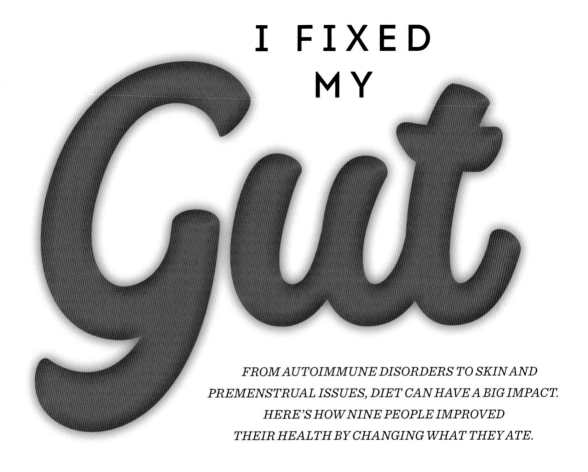

FROM AUTOIMMUNE DISORDERS TO SKIN AND PREMENSTRUAL ISSUES, DIET CAN HAVE A BIG IMPACT. HERE'S HOW NINE PEOPLE IMPROVED THEIR HEALTH BY CHANGING WHAT THEY ATE.

The Problem
Ulcerative Colitis

The summer after college, Gina Foresta, now 51, started having bowel problems, including bloody stools, urgency, pain and more. She was diagnosed at age 23 with ulcerative colitis—a form of inflammatory bowel disease (IBD)—and her doctor told her she'd have to learn to live with it and take medication for the rest of her life. "It was a very doom-and-gloom experience," says Foresta. "I tried different doctors, medications and supplements and took prednisone on and off for years. The side effects of the steroid and other drugs included hair loss, panic attacks, weight gain, bloating and osteopenia [bone loss]."

After struggling for about nine years, Foresta met an osteopathic physician who recommended the Specific Carbohydrate Diet. People with IBD have a hard time digesting di- and polysaccharides, which are types of carbs found in grains, sugars and other foods. "They don't move through the digestive tract quickly enough, so the body responds to them as a foreign agent and the lining becomes inflamed. That's when ulcerations occur and they bleed," says Foresta, who's been on the diet for 20 years now.

GINA FORESTA

"It was like night and day when I went on it. I initially thought there was no way I could do it. I couldn't imagine not eating some carbs, like rice." After being on the diet, she's only had to go on medication a few times in the past 20 years, often as a result of stress or hormonal shifts. "Anything that triggers the immune system can lead to a flare," says Foresta, who uses yoga, exercise and meditation to help manage stress, and makes sure she gets adequate sleep.

The Specific Carbohydrate Diet is similar to the Paleo eating style and since there are so many prepackaged Paleo-friendly foods available now, it's easier to find more things to eat, Foresta says. She uses almond flour instead of wheat flour; avoids all grains, including corn and rice; and eats most vegetables. Since lactose, which is found in dairy, is a disaccharide, she avoids dairy products, except for aged cheeses.

Her gastroenterologist has recommended her diet to some of his patients, and she's helped others try it, too, but because it's so restrictive, it's often a hard sell. "You almost have to hit rock bottom before you give all of that up," she says. "Then you'll wonder why you waited so long to try it. I don't see this way of eating as deprivation; I see it as empowering. I actually have some control over my disease."

The Problem
Lyme Disease

CARLEY SMITH

In 2014, Carley Smith, 33, found herself struggling with health issues. "I just didn't feel like myself. I had my period for four months straight. My tests and blood work came back normal and my doctor told me to go home and put my feet up [to rest]." All the bleeding turned into an infection, and after a stint on antibiotics left her feeling even worse, a friend's prompting made her request a test for Lyme disease, which came back positive.

She started taking medications for it—and then more prescriptions to treat the side effects of the first drugs. "They just seemed to be doing more harm than good," says Smith. "My stomach was so swollen and uncomfortable, I could barely wear pants. When I brought up some information I'd found about gut health and Lyme, my doctor couldn't see any connection."

Smith ultimately came across the Gut and Psychology Syndrome (GAPS) diet. She quit her Lyme medications and started implementing bits and pieces of the diet, like bone broth. "I remember my first sip and it just felt so good to drink," she recalls. "Within a few short weeks I started noticing an improvement. I felt more in control of my body." Eventually she tackled the full elimination and reintroduction phases of the diet. "Within a few months on it, I saw a difference in my energy and mood. The inflammation decreased and I wasn't as sore."

The experience prompted Smith to pursue a Nutritional Therapy Practitioner certification. During that time, though, her mother passed away and Smith suffered a relapse. "My stress levels were through the roof," she recalls. She healed herself again and started Fairy Gutmother (fairygutmother.com), where she works one-on-one with people who are struggling with health issues.

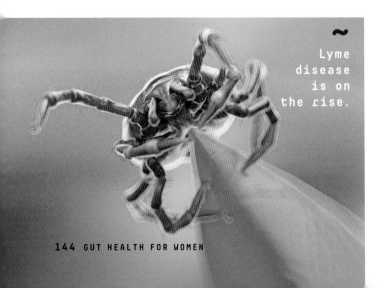

~

Lyme disease is on the rise.

The Problem
Fertility Challenges

Active and seemingly healthy, Anne Harvey and Dan Eigenberg, both 33-year-old educators, decided to change up their diet after experiencing some fertility challenges and a miscarriage in 2019. "After the miscarriage I just wanted to kind of reset my body and feel better," says Harvey. Since inflammation can be a sneaky culprit behind fertility issues, their acupuncturist recommended trying a gut-friendly diet. They considered Paleo, which felt too restrictive, and eventually settled on Whole30. "We approached it like a science experiment," she says.

The couple found books about Whole30 and dove in. "I had days at first where I had headaches and muscle aches and felt listless, but that went away after the first couple of weeks, and then I felt really good," says Eigenberg. Harvey felt better almost immediately. "It was easier to go to the bathroom—I hadn't realized it was an issue—and I had more energy," she says. Her PMS, skin and sleep also improved, and she lost some weight. "I just thought my skin issues were normal, but then they went away with the diet," Harvey adds.

Eigenberg hadn't really paid attention to the uncomfortable bloating and random nausea he'd sometimes experience after eating, until that subsided on the diet. He also noticed that he didn't have as many sinus- and allergy-related issues. "The hard part for me was the lack of carbs on the diet," he says. "I work out six days a week. We ate potatoes but we couldn't eat those 'quick' carbs."

ANNE HARVEY & DAN EIGENBERG

Gut health may impact estrogen levels.

Having each other to rely on made following the diet easier for both of them. "It helped that we both jumped on board and that it was just a month," says Eigenberg. "It would have been harder to do by myself, especially those first few days." Harvey said socializing was particularly difficult on the diet, since they weren't allowed to drink alcohol on the plan "We'd eat beforehand and go out and have water. That was challenging," she recalls. "It was kind of annoying because we talked about it all the time."

After 30 days, the two started slowly adding back foods to see what triggered symptoms; they'd usually notice changes within a few hours. For Harvey, dairy and sugar prompted skin eruptions, and gluten affected her bowel movements. Dairy was a problem for Eigenberg as well and it seemed like bread and gluten products made him feel overly full and nauseated.

After the holidays, the couple, who are still trying to conceive, went back on the diet, at least when they were at home. Says Harvey, "We picked up better habits from doing it. I've discovered that I can easily avoid those things that agitate me and I'd definitely recommend it."

The Problem
SIBO

In 2017, newlywed Emily Sharpe was lying on the bed crying in pain, something that was becoming a frequent occurrence. It felt like someone had punched her in the stomach, and it was just one of many ailments she had suffered with for years, including eczema, hair loss, bloating, extreme allergies, anxiety, exhaustion and constipation. She had been

EMILY SHARPE

~

Sharpe's new hubby coaxed her to finally seek help.

able to tolerate the pain and other symptoms, but her new husband convinced her it wasn't normal.

In the past Sharpe had tried the Whole30 diet, which had helped clear up the eczema and stop the hair loss, so she knew diet was probably key to feeling better. It was during a Paleo f(x) conference, which focused on the popular eating approach, that she first heard about SIBO (small intestinal bacterial overgrowth, for more, see page 46). "I thought, 'I think I have that!'" says Sharpe. "Through the Paleo Physicians Network I looked up a doctor who specialized in gut issues and had experience with SIBO." That doctor prescribed a modified autoimmune Paleo diet, which involved a lot of cooked vegetables, daily bone broth, tons of fiber and no grains, dairy, eggs, legumes, added sugars or nightshades (a group of vegetables, including tomatoes, bell peppers and eggplant, that some people may be sensitive to). She also took glutamine, berberine, oregano oil, magnesium bisglycinate and a probiotic.

Soon, she started sleeping better and had more energy, her eczema almost entirely disappeared and her anxiety decreased.

Sharpe eventually started reintroducing foods. "Figuring out what works is all trial and error," she says. She's added back most nightshades, eggs, oatmeal, quinoa and chickpeas. "I'm entirely off my allergy medications and having regular bowel movements. I don't get as bloated, either." She currently takes a probiotic that includes Bacillus coagulans and Bacillus subtilis. "Don't give up," she advises. "Be your own advocate."

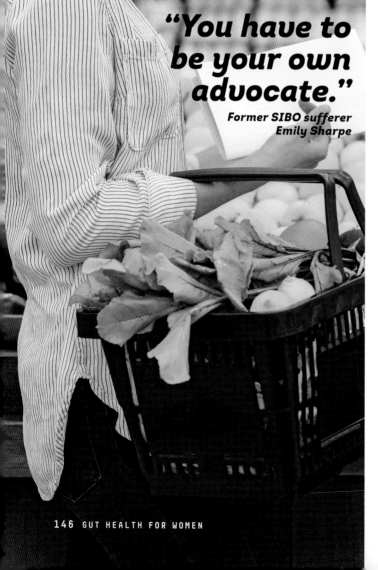

"You have to be your own advocate."
Former SIBO sufferer Emily Sharpe

The Problem
Eczema

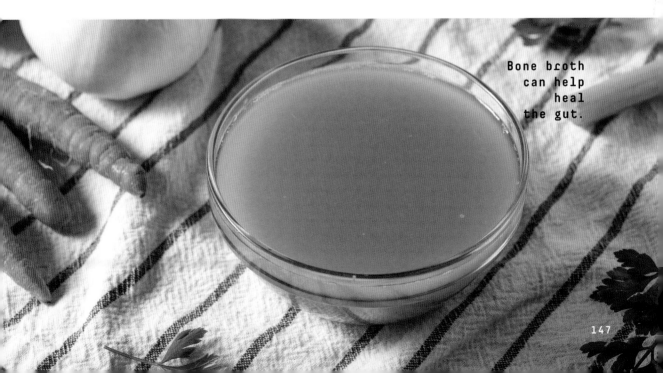

JODY MEAKINS

~

Antibiotics caused Meakins' hard-to-treat eczema.

In 2015, Jody Meakins had been on two courses of antibiotics and, as a result, had suffered two very common but nasty bouts of an infection called Clostridioides difficile—aka "C. diff"—which invades the GI tract (usually after taking antibiotics). "I got over it, but then the eczema showed up," she says. In 2016, during a time when she was also under a lot of stress, she began developing eczema on almost her entire body.

After getting no relief from two dermatologists, Meakins stumbled on a nutrition class at a local rec center, where she found Carley Smith (aka Fairy Gutmother, page 144), a nutrition therapist who specializes in gut issues. "I had done Whole30 before that and it hadn't made a difference, but Carley started me on an even stricter diet specifically designed to heal the gut," says Meakins. "Bone broth was a big part of it and I made my own, either beef or chicken, as well

as my own yogurt. I was trying to make sure everything I ate was as healthy as possible. After three to four months, my skin was completely clear."

Smith put Meakins on the GAPS (Gut and Psychology Syndrome) diet, which eliminates certain foods and then reintroduces them slowly, based on the individual's symptoms. "It's not the foods that are the problem; it's the gut. It has to heal," says Smith.

While the initial diet was strict, Meakins now eats cheese, eggs, oil, butter and meat. "I thought my cholesterol would be sky-high, but it was lower than it had been in years," she says. "Most of it is just cutting out sugar and simple carbs. I also eat a lot of winter squash, which has fiber but is easy to digest."

Meakins says that having patience is key. "You just have to stick to it. If you have a partner or group or an expert to help guide you, it'll be easier to tolerate."

Bone broth can help heal the gut.

The Problem
Weight Gain

A typically active Coloradoan, Kathy Hays, who enjoys hiking, biking and yoga, found herself steadily gaining weight over the years. "No matter what I did or cut out, I was gaining," says Hays, 60. "I craved sweets and also was lacking energy and had migraines, insomnia and chronic stomach issues. When I went to the doctor, he told me I was probably gaining weight because I was getting older."

Hays started taking prescription drugs to help her drop pounds, but it hyped her up and made it more

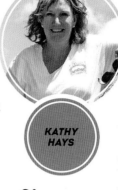

KATHY
HAYS

~

Age does not equal weight gain!

difficult to sleep, so her doctor gave her sleeping pills. Finally, Hays' yoga instructor recommended she contact nutritional therapist Carley Smith. "[Carley] thought I had leaky gut," says Hays. "I started keeping a food diary and found out I was sensitive to gluten and dairy."

Hays shifted her diet to eat more nutrient-dense foods and homemade bone broth ."I was staying away from things like butter and avocado and ghee, but Carley said I need those in my life, so I started adding them in and pairing them with healthy carbs," explains Hays. "She also helped me stop feeling guilty about what I'd eaten when I fell off the wagon."

"Kathy didn't do the full GAPS diet, but we focused on bone broth, cooked foods and adding in some probiotics to help balance her microbiome," says Smith. "She also had a strong craving for sweets, which was probably due to the bacteria or candida, so I had her melt some ghee and honey and put it in a jar. She'd take a spoonful of it every hour in the afternoon to help balance her blood sugar and eliminate cravings."

Over about six months, Hays noticed her energy was returning and her stomach issues were completely gone. Today, she rarely has a migraine, is sleeping better, and has lost about 20 pounds. In addition, she's no longer taking any prescription medications. "I feel like I'm just getting better and stronger and younger every day!" says Hays,who adds she has as much energy as when she was in her 20s and 30s. What I've learned is it's all tied to your gut. I'd be looking at that first for any kind of health concerns—and don't buy it when they try to put you on pharmaceuticals. Look at your diet."

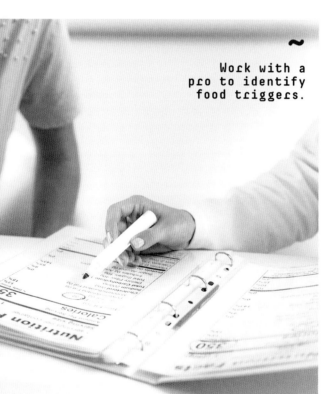

~

Work with a pro to identify food triggers.

The Problem
Celiac

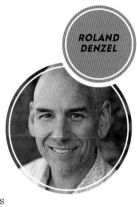

Small for her age and a late bloomer, Jesse Shroyer, 34, started having GI symptoms—she'd get sick after eating—as a teen. Doctors removed her gallbladder at age 17 and she felt better, but she suffered with IBS throughout college. After graduation, frequent travel and a high-stress job prompted a return of her symptoms. "The first time it happened, I thought I had food poisoning," she recalls. "Then I started getting brain fog, acne and cavities, and having extreme nausea and constipation."

In 2012, a test for celiac disease came back positive and a nutritionist helped her cut out the obvious (grains such as wheat, rye and barley) and less obvious (some spices, soy sauce and oats) sources of gluten. She also started taking a mild antidepressant for anxiety. "My gut was so compromised, anything that was even slightly cross-contaminated [like oats] would send me to the bathroom for hours," she says. "I was having panic attacks."

Five years later, stress triggered another outbreak and a doctor told her she had two parasites and an overgrowth of E. coli and candida.

An elimination diet that cut out dairy, corn, soy, sugar, caffeine, alcohol and peanuts helped her pinpoint triggering foods, and she also started supplementing with curcumin, an anti-inflammatory, among other things. "On day eight of the diet I woke up feeling like a different person. I had energy and no stomach issues or joint pain," she remembers. Recent imaging shows her gut still hasn't fully healed so Shroyer has cut out all grains and dairy. She also teaches yoga, meditates and journals to help manage stress.

~
Stress can bring on a relapse

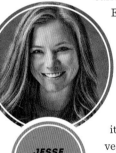

JESSE SHROYER

The Problem
Headaches

After losing 110 pounds in 2002, Roland Denzel thought he was pretty fit. In 2008, while he was no longer struggling with his weight, he'd noticed that he was getting daily headaches. He'd had migraines as a child, and they had subsided for the most part. The newer headaches had gotten to the point that he was carrying small resealable bags of ibuprofen wherever he went. "I had them stashed everywhere—my computer bag, my glove compartment. If I didn't take four to six pills a day when I got a headache, it would get worse and I'd have to go lie down," he recalls.

Denzel, 52, cut out alcohol and caffeine for 30 days, but it didn't help. Eventually, he heard about the Paleo diet. "I initially thought it was too extreme, but then I thought, why not try it for a while," he recalls. "I didn't even call it Paleo; I just tried to focus on eating whole foods. I cut out higher-sugar items and dairy, beans, legumes, and vegetable and seed oils." Denzel didn't realize the headaches were gone until a couple of months later when he stumbled across a bag of ibuprofen in his computer bag. "That's when I realized I hadn't needed them." Denzel, who's now a health coach, also noticed that although the scale hadn't budged on the diet, his clothes fit better because he wasn't as bloated.

He has reintroduced most foods, but in smaller amounts. "I eat rice and corn almost every day, but not at every meal," says Denzel. "If I eat more things at a higher level, like a lot of grains, I'll notice my scalp starts to get itchier and I get more headaches."

ROLAND DENZEL

~
A Paleo-ish diet spelled relief.

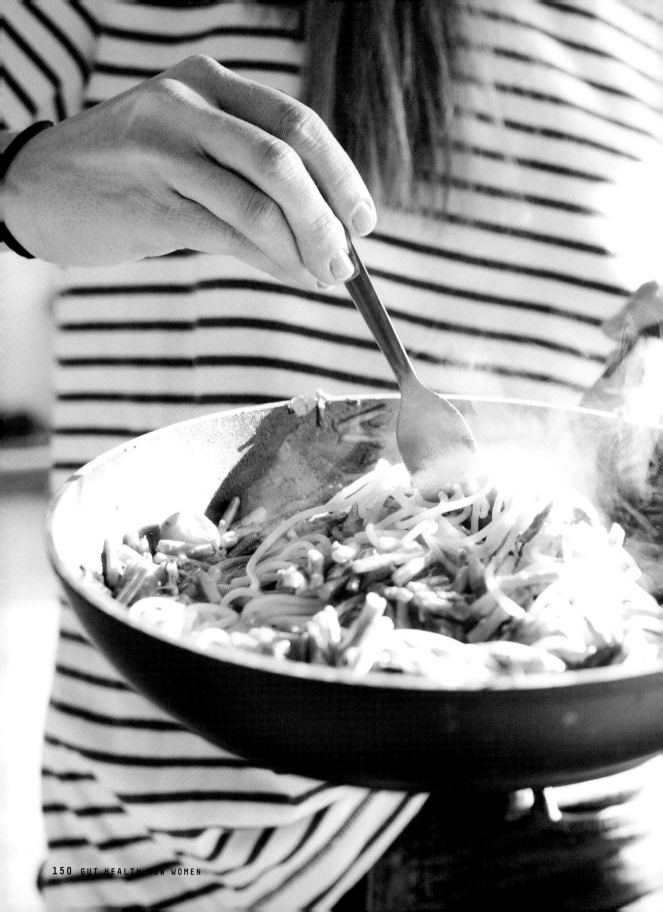

5

Recipes

READY TO START IMPROVING FROM THE INSIDE OUT?
HERE ARE DOZENS OF IDEAS FOR DELICIOUS DISHES THAT
WILL MAKE YOUR MOUTH—AND MICROBIOME—HAPPY.

Breakfast

IT'S NEVER TOO EARLY IN THE DAY TO WORK ON YOUR GUT HEALTH. WHETHER YOU LIKE YOUR BREAKFAST LIGHT AND FRUITY, OR PREFER SOMETHING HEARTIER AND PROTEIN-PACKED, YOU'LL FIND PLENTY OF OPTIONS HERE.

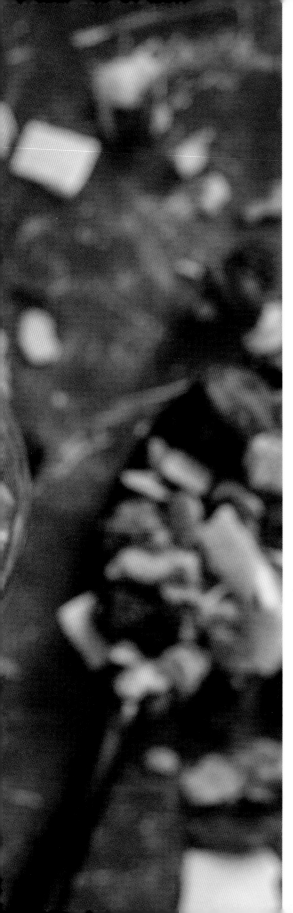

Coconut Granola With Pumpkin Seeds and Dried Fruits

Easy—Kid Friendly—Vegan

Coconut contains good-for-you fats and disease-fighting antioxidants. Enjoy this granola with coconut milk, or top with yogurt for extra protein.

PREP *10 minutes*

TOTAL *30 minutes*

SERVINGS *10*

Ingredients

- ½ cup honey
- ½ teaspoon cinnamon
- ½ cup coconut oil
- 3 cups old-fashioned rolled oats
- ½ cup chopped walnuts
- ½ cup pepitas (pumpkin seeds)
- ⅓ cup toasted coconut flakes
- ⅓ cup goji berries
- ⅓ cup dried blueberries

Instructions

1 Preheat oven to 300°F. Line a rimmed baking sheet with parchment paper and set aside.

2 In a large bowl, whisk together honey, cinnamon and oil.

3 Stir in oats, walnuts and pumpkin seeds.

4 Spread mixture evenly on baking sheet.

5 Bake for 20 minutes, stirring halfway through.

6 Remove from oven and stir in coconut flakes, goji berries and blueberries.

7 Store in an airtight container at room temperature.

Asparagus and Avocado Toast With Hard-Boiled Eggs

Easy—Vegetarian

Asparagus is a low-calorie vegetable that is high in antioxidants and is an excellent source of folate and vitamins A, C and K.

PREP *5 minutes*

TOTAL *15 minutes*

SERVINGS *4*

Ingredients

- 2 avocados, halved and pitted
- ½ teaspoon sea salt
- 1 teaspoon lime juice
- 4 slices crusty sourdough bread, toasted
- 20 thin asparagus spears, trimmed and steamed
- 4 hard-boiled eggs, sliced
- 2 teaspoons Aleppo pepper
- 4 tablespoons microgreens or watercress

Instructions

1 In a small bowl, mash avocado with salt and lime juice.

2 Spread mixture evenly over the 4 toast pieces.

3 Top each toast with 5 asparagus spears and then with sliced eggs.

4 Sprinkle evenly with Aleppo pepper and microgreens to serve.

Microgreens add color and nutrients.

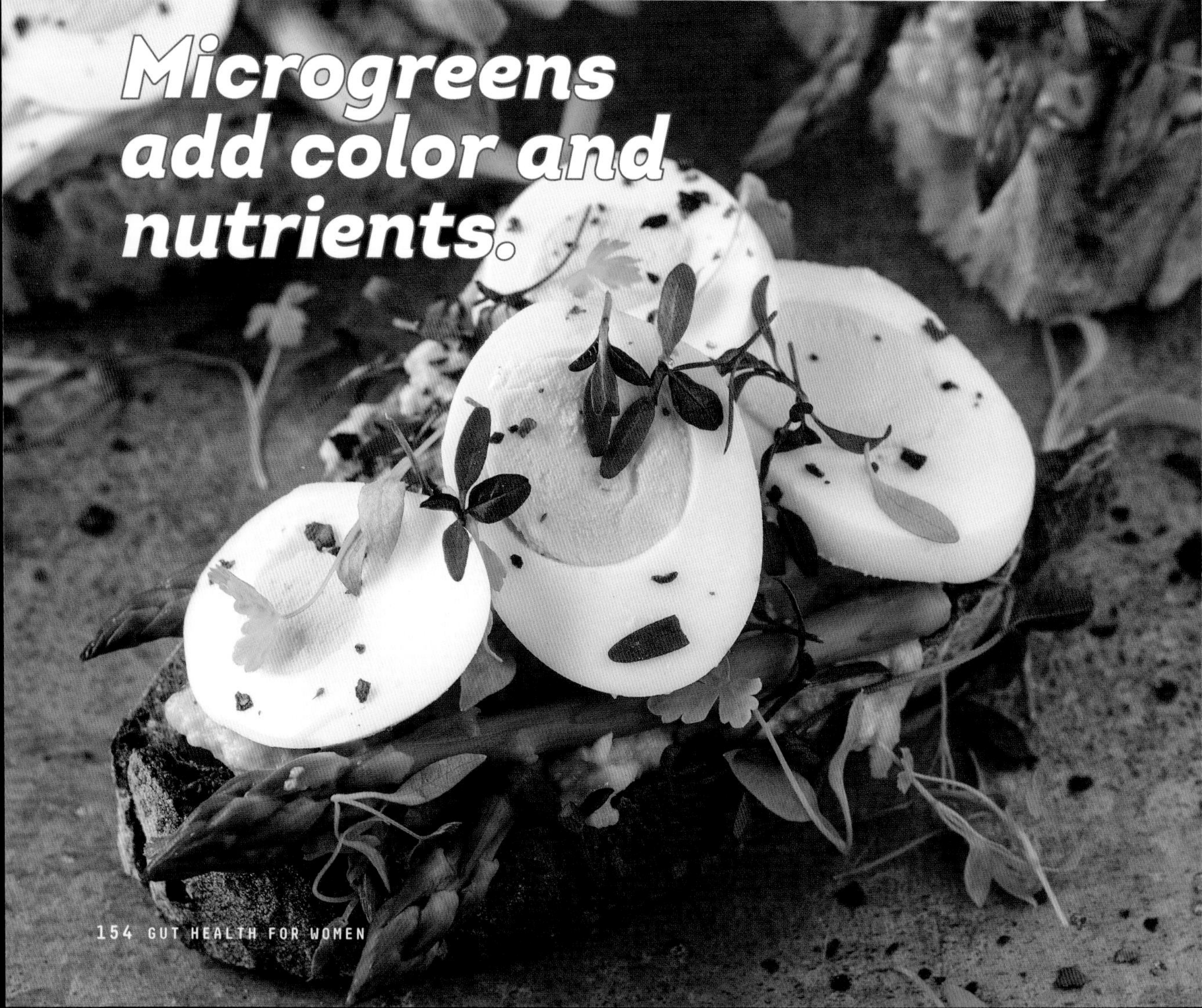

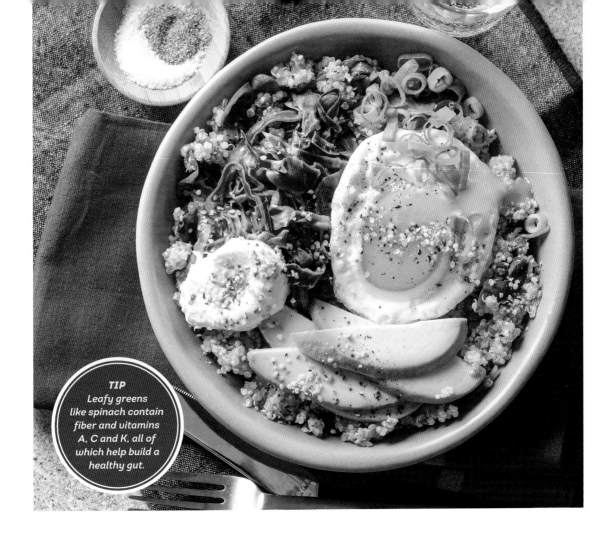

TIP
Leafy greens like spinach contain fiber and vitamins A, C and K, all of which help build a healthy gut.

Probiotic Breakfast Bowl

Easy—Gluten Free—Vegetarian

Probiotics are bacteria that provide powerful health benefits. They aid in making food more digestible, which in turn increases your gut's ability to absorb vitamins and minerals.

PREP *10 minutes*

TOTAL *30 minutes*

SERVINGS *4*

Ingredients

- 1 cup uncooked quinoa
- 2 cups vegetable broth
- ½ teaspoon sea salt
- 2 cups baby spinach leaves
- 4 fried eggs
- 2 avocados, sliced
- 3 green onions, sliced
- 1 cup fermented purplecabbage or kimchi
- ¼ cup plain Greek yogurt
- 4 teaspoons hemp seeds

Instructions

1 In a medium saucepan, combine quinoa, broth and salt. Bring to a boil.

2 Cover, reduce heat and simmer 15 minutes or until liquid is absorbed.

3 Remove from heat, stir in spinach, cover and let stand 5 minutes.

4 Fluff with a fork and divide evenly among 4 bowls.

5 Top each bowl with a fried egg and equal amounts of avocado slices, green onion slices, fermented cabbage, yogurt and hemp seeds.

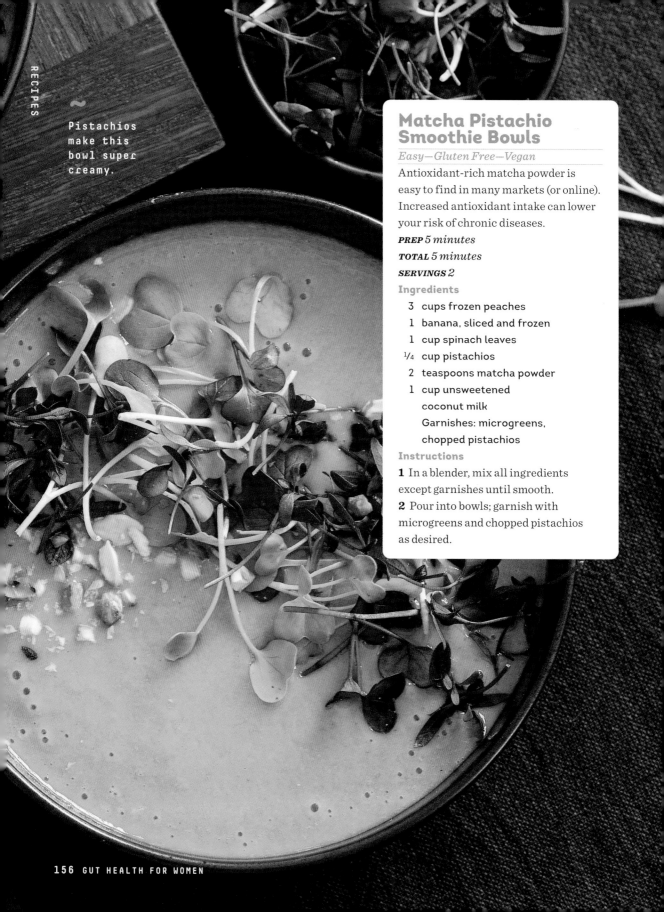

~ Pistachios make this bowl super creamy.

Matcha Pistachio Smoothie Bowls

Easy—Gluten Free—Vegan

Antioxidant-rich matcha powder is easy to find in many markets (or online). Increased antioxidant intake can lower your risk of chronic diseases.

PREP *5 minutes*

TOTAL *5 minutes*

SERVINGS *2*

Ingredients

- 3 cups frozen peaches
- 1 banana, sliced and frozen
- 1 cup spinach leaves
- 1/4 cup pistachios
- 2 teaspoons matcha powder
- 1 cup unsweetened coconut milk
- Garnishes: microgreens, chopped pistachios

Instructions

1 In a blender, mix all ingredients except garnishes until smooth.

2 Pour into bowls; garnish with microgreens and chopped pistachios as desired.

High fiber, high flavor—a win-win!

Blueberry Almond Smoothie

Easy—Gluten Free—Vegetarian

Freeze banana slices for at least an hour before blending this smoothie; the freezing (and the oatmeal) makes it extra thick.

PREP *5 minutes*

TOTAL *5 minutes*

SERVINGS *2*

Ingredients

- 2 cups unsweetened almond milk
- 1½ cups frozen blueberries
- 2 large bananas, sliced and frozen
- ¼ cup almond butter
- 1 cup old-fashioned oats
- 2 tablespoons honey
  Garnishes: sugarcane swizzle stick, blueberries, mint sprig

Instructions

1 In a blender, mix all ingredients except garnishes until smooth.

2 Pour into glass; garnish as desired.

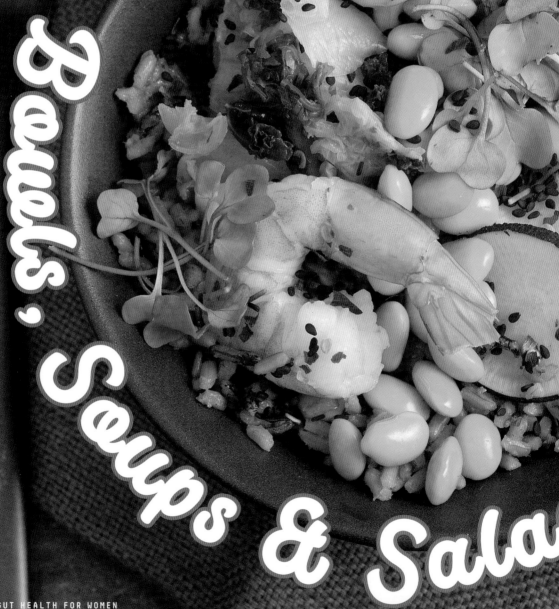

WHETHER IT'S LUNCH OR DINNER, APPETIZER OR MINI MEAL, THESE LIGHTER DISHES ARE STILL CHOCK-FULL OF NUTRIENTS TO NOURISH YOUR WHOLE BODY.

Bowls, Soups & Salads

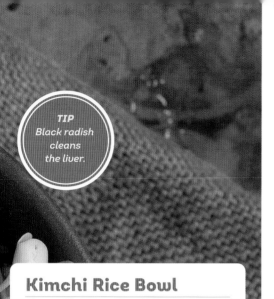

TIP
Black radish
cleans
the liver.

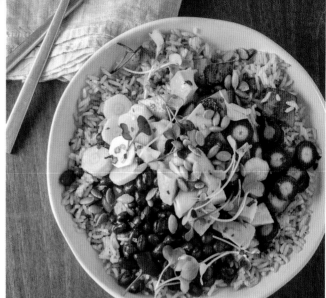

Kimchi Rice Bowl

Easy—Gluten Free—Vegetarian

Edamame is an excellent source of
protein and other nutrients, while
kimchi—like most fermented foods—
helps promote a healthy microbiome.

PREP *5 minutes*

TOTAL *10 minutes*

SERVINGS *2*

Ingredients

- 1 (8.5-ounce) package precooked
  brown rice/wild rice medley,
  microwaved according to package
  directions
- 1 cup kimchi
- 4 jumbo shrimp, cooked
- ½ cup cooked edamame
- ¼ cup black radish slices
- ¼ cup radish microgreens
- ¼ cup rice wine vinegar
  Garnishes: black sesame seeds,
  red pepper flakes

Instructions

1 Divide rice evenly between
2 individual serving bowls.

2 Top each bowl with half of kimchi,
shrimp, edamame, radish and
microgreens.

3 Sprinkle each bowl with rice wine
vinegar; top with sesame seeds and
red pepper flakes as desired.

Power Bowl

Easy—Vegetarian

Butternut squash is full of vitamins, minerals and
antioxidants as well as fiber. Carrots add color and
crunch to this gut-friendly dish, in addition to
beta-carotene and potassium.

PREP *15 minutes*

TOTAL *15 minutes*

SERVINGS *2*

Ingredients

- 1 (8-ounce) microwavable bag turmeric rice,
  cooked according to package directions
- 1 (15-ounce) can black beans,
  drained and rinsed
- 1 cup cubed and cooked butternut squash
- 1 small yellow carrot, sliced
- 1 small purple carrot, sliced
- 1 small avocado, coarsely chopped
- ¼ cup roasted pepitas
- ¼ teaspoon red pepper flakes
  Garnish: radish microgreens

Instructions

1 Divide the cooked turmeric rice between
2 individual serving bowls.

2 Evenly top with black beans, squash, carrots,
avocado, pepitas and red pepper flakes.

3 Garnish with radish microgreens as desired.

Mexican Grain Bowl With Red Beans, Corn and Tomatoes

Easy—Gluten Free—Vegan

Quinoa is gluten-free, high in protein and fiber and contains all nine essential amino acids.

PREP *15 minutes*

TOTAL *15 minutes*

SERVINGS *2*

Ingredients

- 1 (8.5-ounce) bag microwavable organic quinoa, brown and red rice with flaxseed, cooked according to package directions
- ½ teaspoon sea salt
- ¼ teaspoon ground black pepper
- 1 (15-ounce) can red beans, drained and rinsed
- 1 pint cherry tomatoes, halved
- 1 ear of corn, scraped
- 1 small purple onion, sliced
  Garnishes: jalapeño pepper slices, Fresno pepper slices, lime slices

Instructions

1 In a medium bowl, mix cooked quinoa and rice mixture, salt and pepper. Divide mixture between 2 individual serving bowls.

2 Evenly divide beans, tomatoes, corn and onion slices between bowls.

3 Top with desired garnishes.

Beans add fiber and nutrients.

TIP
If you've got leftover cooked tofu, tempeh or seitan, add it to this bowl.

M

Citrus Chicken Salad Bowl

Easy—Kid Friendly

This colorful meal makes a tasty lunch to pack for the office or school.

PREP *10 minutes*

TOTAL *15 minutes*

SERVINGS *2*

Ingredients

- 1 (8-ounce) bag organic fully cooked coconut rice
- 1 cup chicken breast, sliced
- ½ cup chopped celery
- 1 small orange, sectioned
- 1 cup purple cabbage, thinly sliced
- ½ cup pea sprouts
- 1 tablespoon hot sesame oil
- 1 tablespoon tamari
- ⅛ teaspoon red pepper flakes
  Garnishes: lime wedges, red pepper flakes

Instructions

1 Heat coconut rice according to package directions.

2 Divide rice evenly between 2 individual serving bowls.

3 Top each with half of the chicken, celery, orange, cabbage and pea sprouts.

4 In a small bowl, whisk together hot sesame oil, tamari and red pepper flakes.

5 Drizzle mixture over bowls.

6 Garnish with lime wedges and red pepper flakes as desired.

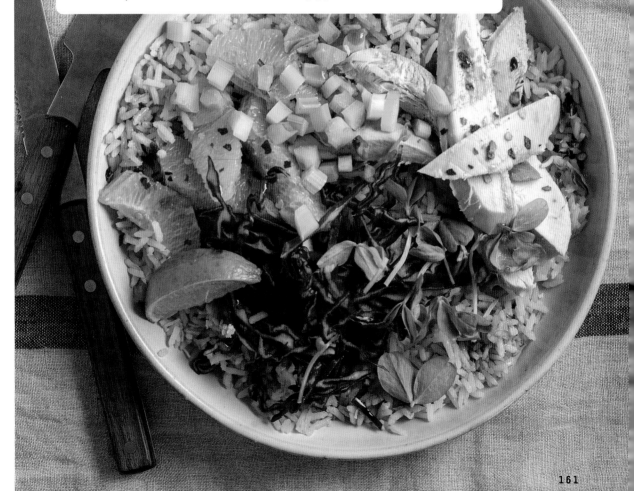

Chicken Bone Broth

Easy—Gluten Free

Made in a slow cooker, this broth is flavorful and rich. Use cooked chicken bones if you've got any left from a roasted chicken. It will elevate any recipe that calls for chicken broth, and it's delicious on its own. Broth will keep in the fridge for five days; freeze for longer storage.

PREP *5 minutes*

TOTAL *10 minutes,*

+ 1 day inactive

SERVINGS *24*

Ingredients

- 3 pounds raw chicken bones
- 1 large onion, coarsely chopped
- 1 tablespoon apple cider vinegar
- 1 tablespoon minced garlic
- 1 tablespoon sea salt
- 4 fresh bay leaves
- 3 quarts water

Garnish: chopped parsley

Instructions

1 In the pot of a slow cooker, combine bones, onion, vinegar, garlic, salt and bay leaves. Cover with water, stopping at least 1 inch from top of pot.

2 Place lid on slow cooker; cook on low for 24 hours.

3 With a slotted spoon, remove and discard solids.

4 Pour mixture through a strainer; let cool.

5 Transfer to three 1-quart glass jars with lids; store in refrigerator.

6 Garnish with parsley when serving.

Bone broth is full of nutrients.

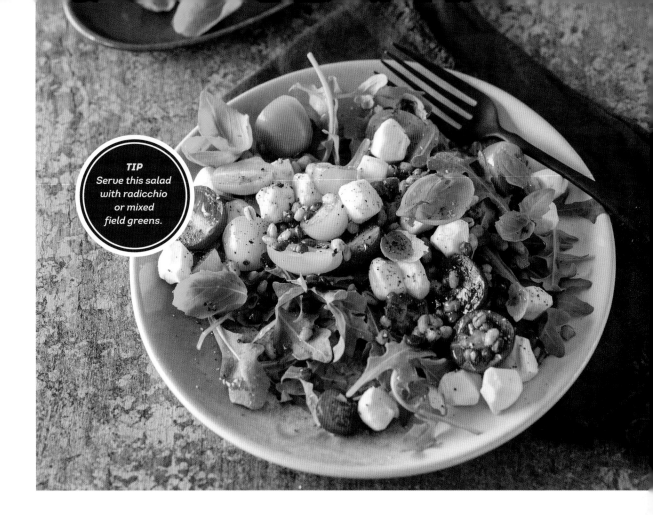

TIP
Serve this salad with radicchio or mixed field greens.

Caprese Barley and Green Lentil Salad

Easy—Vegetarian

Barley has several impressive gut health benefits, particularly its high soluble-fiber content, which is believed to help lower blood pressure and LDL ("bad") cholesterol. The whole grain also contains protein, iron and selenium.

PREP *5 minutes*

TOTAL *10 minutes*

SERVINGS *4*

Ingredients

- 1 (8.8-ounce) microwavable bag barley and green lentils, cooked according to package directions
- 1 pint multicolored cherry tomatoes, halved
- 1 (8-ounce) container pearl mozzarella, drained
- ¼ cup olive oil
- 2 tablespoons red wine vinegar
- 1 tablespoon Dijon mustard
- ¼ teaspoon sea salt
- ¼ teaspoon ground black pepper
  Garnishes: basil leaves, micro radish greens

Instructions

1 In a large bowl, combine barley mixture, tomatoes and mozzarella.

2 In a blender, mix olive oil, vinegar, mustard, salt and pepper until smooth to make dressing.

3 Pour dressing over barley mixture; toss to combine.

4 Garnish as desired before serving.

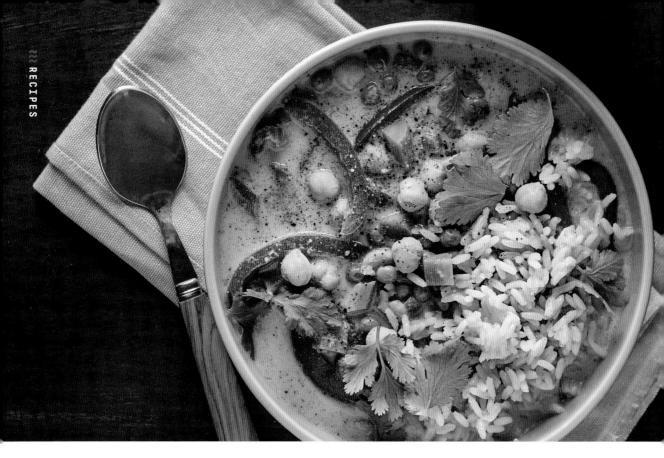

Thai Green Curry Soup

Easy—Gluten Free—Vegan

Turmeric, lemongrass and ginger all
stimulate digestion; they also give this
soup a delightful fragrance.

PREP *10 minutes*

TOTAL *40 minutes*

SERVINGS *4*

Ingredients

2 tablespoons coconut oil

1 teaspoon minced garlic

1 cup sliced green onions

2 stalks lemongrass, diced

3 carrots, diced

1 tablespoon minced ginger

3 tablespoons chopped basil

2 tablespoons green curry paste

1 teaspoon ground turmeric

1 (15-ounce) can chickpeas, drained and rinsed

1 (15-ounce) can coconut milk

1 cup vegetable broth

1 tablespoon tamari

2 tablespoons lime juice

1 teaspoon salt

1 red bell pepper, sliced

1 cup frozen green peas

Cooked brown rice

Garnishes: cilantro sprigs,
green onions

Instructions

1 In a Dutch oven over medium-high heat, heat oil.
Add garlic, green onion, lemongrass, carrots,
ginger and basil.

2 Cook for 4 to 5 minutes. Stir in green curry paste
and turmeric; cook for 1 minute.

3 Add chickpeas, coconut milk, broth, tamari, lime
juice, salt and bell pepper.

4 Simmer for 10 to 15 minutes; stir in peas
to heat through.

5 Serve over brown rice; garnish as desired.

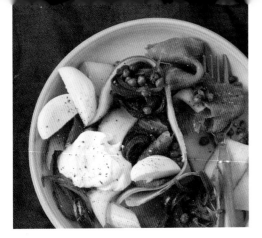

Smoked Salmon Salad With Cucumber Ribbons and Red Onion

Easy—Gluten Free—Vegetarian

Pickled onions and gut-healthy yogurt add a nice tartness to this dish.

PREP *10 minutes*

TOTAL *15 minutes,*
+ 15 minutes inactive

SERVINGS *4*

Ingredients

- 1 small red onion, thinly sliced
- 1 cup red wine vinegar
- 1 tablespoon sugar
- ½ teaspoon salt
- 1½ teaspoons dried dill
- 1 (8-ounce) package smoked salmon
- 1 English cucumber, skin on, sliced into ribbons
- 2 hard-boiled eggs, quartered
- ¼ cup Greek yogurt
  Cracked black pepper
  Garnish: capers

Instructions

1 In a small saucepan over medium-high heat, add red onion, vinegar, sugar, salt and dried dill. Bring to a boil. Cover and let stand about 15 minutes.

2 On a large platter, arrange salmon pieces, cucumber ribbons, eggs and dollops of yogurt. Drain onion mixture and place on top.

3 Top with cracked pepper and capers just before serving.

Kale Caesar Salad With Garlic Roasted Chickpeas

Easy—Gluten Free—Vegan

Raw or cooked, kale is the king of the supergreens. Tahini is full of good fats and may reduce inflammation.

PREP *5 minutes*

TOTAL *15 minutes*

SERVINGS *4*

Ingredients

- ½ cup olive oil
- 2 tablespoons lemon juice
- 2 tablespoons tahini
- 1 tablespoon Dijon mustard
- 1 teaspoon minced garlic
- ¼ teaspoon sea salt
- 1 (15-ounce) can chickpeas, drained and rinsed
- 1 teaspoon garlic salt
- 1 teaspoon ground black pepper
- 4 cups chopped kale leaves
  Garnish: lemon wedges

Instructions

1 In a blender add olive oil, lemon juice, tahini, mustard, garlic and sea salt; blend until smooth. Set aside.

2 In a large skillet over medium heat, add chickpeas, garlic salt and pepper. Toast for 5 minutes or until chickpeas begin to dry out.

3 Divide kale evenly between 4 plates; drizzle with dressing and sprinkle with chickpeas.

4 Garnish with lemon wedges.

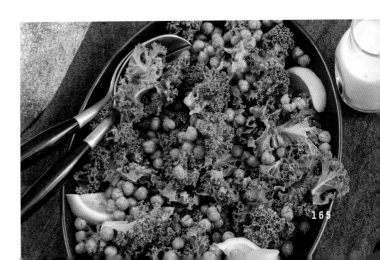

THESE SAVORY MAIN DISHES SUIT A VARIETY OF DIETS AND TASTES. WHAT DO THEY ALL HAVE IN COMMON? INGREDIENTS AND SEASONINGS THAT KEEP YOUR GUT HEALTHY.

Entrees

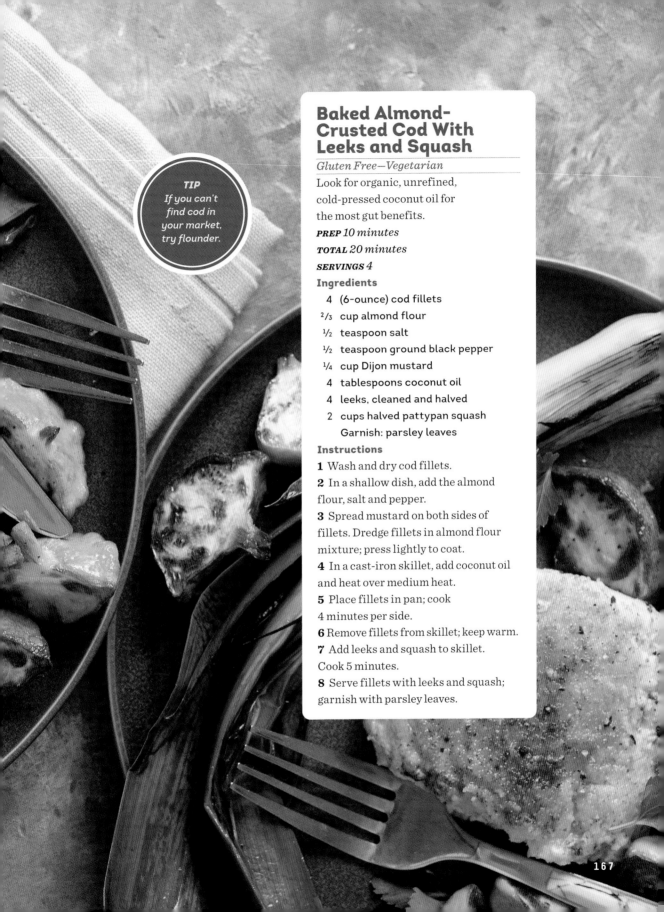

TIP
If you can't find cod in your market, try flounder.

Baked Almond-Crusted Cod With Leeks and Squash

Gluten Free—Vegetarian

Look for organic, unrefined, cold-pressed coconut oil for the most gut benefits.

PREP *10 minutes*

TOTAL *20 minutes*

SERVINGS *4*

Ingredients

- 4 (6-ounce) cod fillets
- ²/₃ cup almond flour
- ½ teaspoon salt
- ½ teaspoon ground black pepper
- ¼ cup Dijon mustard
- 4 tablespoons coconut oil
- 4 leeks, cleaned and halved
- 2 cups halved pattypan squash
  Garnish: parsley leaves

Instructions

1 Wash and dry cod fillets.

2 In a shallow dish, add the almond flour, salt and pepper.

3 Spread mustard on both sides of fillets. Dredge fillets in almond flour mixture; press lightly to coat.

4 In a cast-iron skillet, add coconut oil and heat over medium heat.

5 Place fillets in pan; cook 4 minutes per side.

6 Remove fillets from skillet; keep warm.

7 Add leeks and squash to skillet. Cook 5 minutes.

8 Serve fillets with leeks and squash; garnish with parsley leaves.

Simple, fresh and healthy!

Cherry Tomato and Roasted Garlic Pasta

Easy—Gluten Free—Vegetarian

Caramelizing the tomatoes and garlic together really brings out their flavors.

PREP *20 minutes*

TOTAL *35 minutes*

SERVINGS *4*

Ingredients

- 1 (12-ounce) box organic brown rice gluten-free capellini pasta
- 1 (12-ounce) package multicolored cherry tomatoes, halved
- 2 tablespoons olive oil
- ½ teaspoon salt
- ½ teaspoon ground black pepper
- 1 teaspoon chopped garlic
  Garnishes: oregano leaves, grated Parmesan

Instructions

1 Cook pasta according to package directions.

2 Preheat oven to 300°F.

3 Meanwhile, on a large rimmed baking sheet, toss together tomatoes, olive oil, salt, pepper and garlic.

4 Roast until tomatoes are caramelized, about 15 minutes.

5 Toss pasta and tomatoes together.

6 Serve in bowls; garnish as desired.

Grilled Pork Tenderloin and Snap Peas

Easy—Gluten Free—Kid Friendly

Sugar snap peas have lots of fiber, which can help your digestive system run smoothly.

PREP *10 minutes*

TOTAL *30 minutes,*
+ 10 minutes inactive

SERVINGS *4*

Ingredients

- 1   pound pork tenderloin
- ½   teaspoon granulated garlic
- ½   teaspoon salt
- ½   teaspoon ground black pepper
- 1   tablespoon olive oil
- 1   (8-ounce) bag sugar snap peas, cooked
- 1   (8.5-ounce) bag red quinoa and brown rice, cooked according to package directions

  Garnish: pea shoots

Instructions

1 Sprinkle all surfaces of pork tenderloin with granulated garlic, salt and pepper.

2 Brush grill pan with olive oil; place over medium-high heat.

3 Grill pork for 18 minutes, turning occasionally, until cooked through.

4 Remove pork from grill; let rest on a cutting board for 10 minutes. Slice into medallions.

5 Divide peas and quinoa mixture evenly between 4 dinner plates; top with pork medallions and garnish with pea shoots as desired.

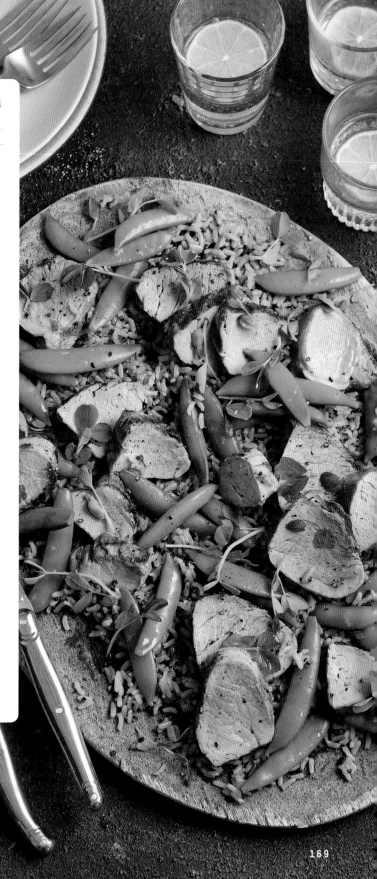

Sesame Garlic Chicken With Broccolini

Gluten Free—Kid Friendly

Broccolini is a tender cross between broccoli and Chinese broccoli; it adds an earthy, slightly sweet taste (and great gut benefits) to this dish.

PREP *5 minutes*

TOTAL *15 minutes*

SERVINGS *4*

Ingredients

- 1 tablespoon sesame oil
- 1 tablespoon chili oil
- 4 boneless, skinless chicken breasts, cubed
- ½ teaspoon salt
- ¼ teaspoon ground black pepper
- 1 (8.8-ounce) package precooked rice, microwaved according to package directions
- 1 (8-ounce) package Broccolini, cooked according to package directions
- ¼ cup cooked edamame
- 1 (12-ounce) bottle garlic-chili sauce
  Garnish: red pepper flakes

Instructions

1 In a skillet over medium-high heat, add sesame and chili oils.

2 Sprinkle chicken evenly with salt and pepper. Add chicken to skillet; cook, stirring constantly, for 6 minutes.

3 Meanwhile, divide warm rice evenly between 4 individual serving bowls. Top with cooked chicken, Broccolini and edamame. Drizzle with garlic-chili sauce and garnish with red pepper flakes as desired.

Garlicky Sauteed Shrimp

Easy—Gluten Free—Kid Friendly

Garlic lovers rejoice: It's a healthy prebiotic, so add as much as you'd like to these tasty shrimp.

PREP *5 minutes*

TOTAL *10 minutes*

SERVINGS *4*

Ingredients

- 1 pound large raw shrimp (31-35 count per pound), peeled and deveined
- 3 cloves garlic, chopped
- 2 tablespoons avocado oil
- ¼ teaspoon salt
- ¼ teaspoon ground black pepper
- 2 green onions, sliced
- Garnish: lemon wedges

Instructions

1 In a large bowl, toss shrimp, garlic, oil, salt and pepper to coat.

2 In a cast-iron skillet over medium-high heat, add shrimp mixture. Cook for 4 minutes or until shrimp is no longer opaque.

3 Remove shrimp from skillet and serve; garnish with lemon wedges.

TIP
Serve these shrimp with rice and sauteed spinach.

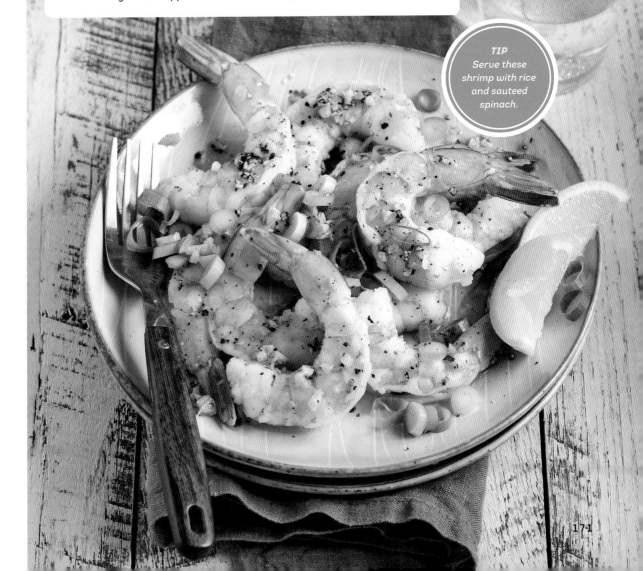

~

Serve this dip with a rainbow of colorful crudité.

LOOKING FOR A NEW SIDE DISH TO SERVE WITH DINNER TONIGHT? OR MAYBE A LITTLE SOMETHING TO OFFER AT A PARTY? KEEP IT DELICIOUS— AND HEALTHY—WITH THESE RECIPES.

Snacks &

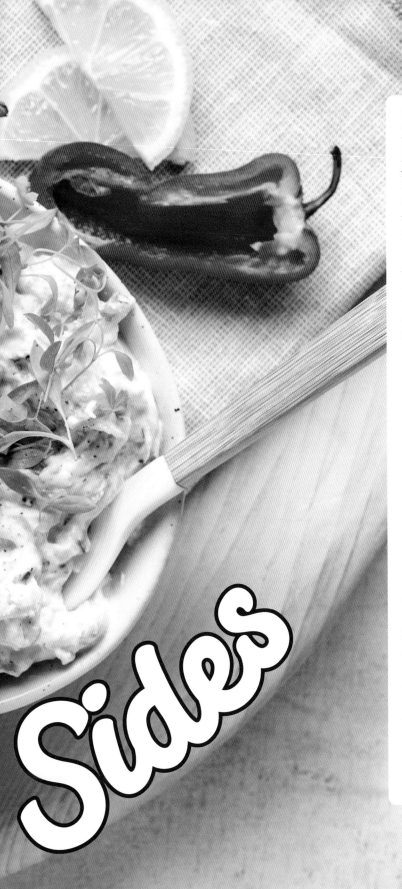

Mediterranean Zucchini Dip With Mini Peppers

Kid Friendly—Vegetarian

Zucchini helps improve digestion and contains significant fiber, which is key for a healthy gut. This dip is thick enough to spread on crackers or pita chips, too.

PREP *10 minutes*

TOTAL *20 minutes,*
+ 30 minutes inactive

SERVINGS *4*

Ingredients

- 1 tablespoon coconut oil
- 2 zucchini, grated
- ¼ cup diced sweet onion
- 1 teaspoon minced garlic
- ½ teaspoon salt
- ¼ teaspoon pepper
- ¼ teaspoon cumin
- 1 tablespoon lemon juice
- 1 teaspoon lemon zest
- 1 tablespoon chopped herbs (basil, mint, parsley, dill, oregano)
- ⅓ cup plain Greek yogurt
  Garnish: micro parsley
  Mini sweet peppers, halved

Instructions

1 In a skillet over medium-high heat, heat oil. Add zucchini, onion, garlic, salt and pepper.

2 Saute for 10 minutes.

3 Stir in cumin, lemon juice and zest.

4 Let cool for 30 minutes.

5 In a serving bowl, mix cooled vegetables, herbs and yogurt; garnish with parsley.

6 Serve with mini peppers.

Sides

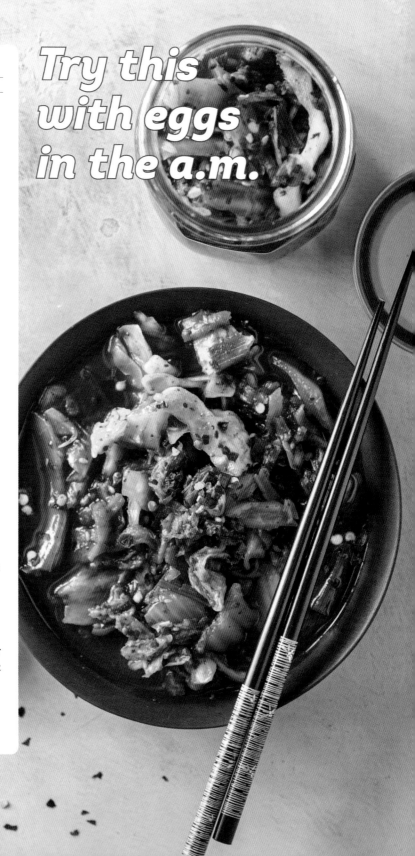

Kimchi

Easy—Gluten Free—Vegetarian

The longer this kimchi sits in the refrigerator, the better and more intense the flavor will be.

PREP *15 minutes*

TOTAL *15 minutes,*
+ 13 hours inactive

SERVINGS *8*

Ingredients

- 1 head napa cabbage, sliced
- 1 tablespoon sea salt
- 1 teaspoon minced garlic
- 1 teaspoon grated ginger
- 1 tablespoon fish sauce
- 2 tablespoons garlic chili sauce
- 3 tablespoons rice vinegar
- ¼ cup matchstick carrots
- 1 small onion, sliced
- ¼ cup sliced green onion
- 1 teaspoon sesame seeds

Instructions

1 In a large bowl, place cabbage; sprinkle with sea salt and set aside for 1 hour.

2 Meanwhile, in a small bowl, mix garlic, ginger, fish sauce, garlic chili sauce and vinegar.

3 Rinse cabbage under water; drain and dry thoroughly. Return to large bowl.

4 Toss in garlic mixture; stir in carrots, onion, green onion and sesame seeds.

5 Place kimchi in a large glass jar with lid; seal and leave to ferment at room temperature overnight, then place in refrigerator.

6 Kimchi will keep in the refrigerator for 2 weeks.

Try this with eggs in the a.m.

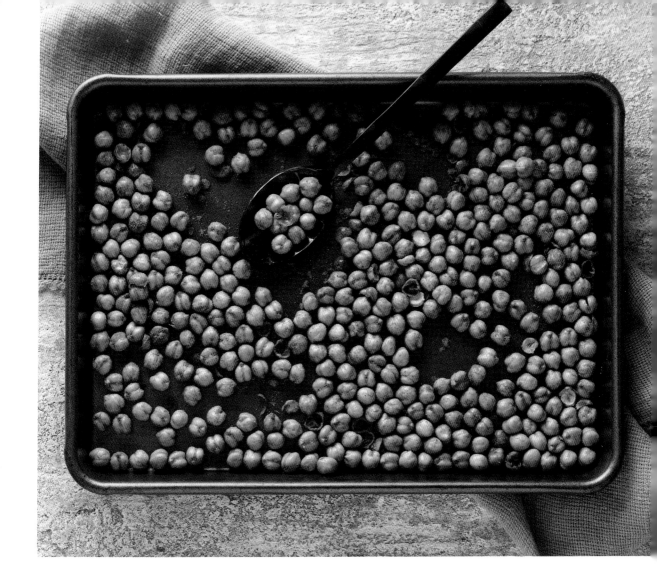

Smoky Baked Chickpeas

Easy—Gluten Free—Vegan

Chickpeas are full of protein and
soluble fiber, which helps increase the
amount of healthy bacteria in your gut.
Double this recipe for a party.

PREP *5 minutes*

TOTAL *30 minutes*

SERVINGS *4*

Ingredients

1 (15-ounce) can chickpeas,
  drained and rinsed

1 tablespoon vegetable oil

1 teaspoon chili powder

½ teaspoon cayenne pepper

½ teaspoon smoked paprika

½ teaspoon cumin

Instructions

1 Preheat oven to 425°F. Cover a baking sheet
with parchment paper.

2 Toss chickpeas with oil and seasonings.
Spread on baking sheet.

3 Bake for 25 minutes or until crunchy.

4 Let cool completely.

5 Store in an airtight container for up to
2 weeks.

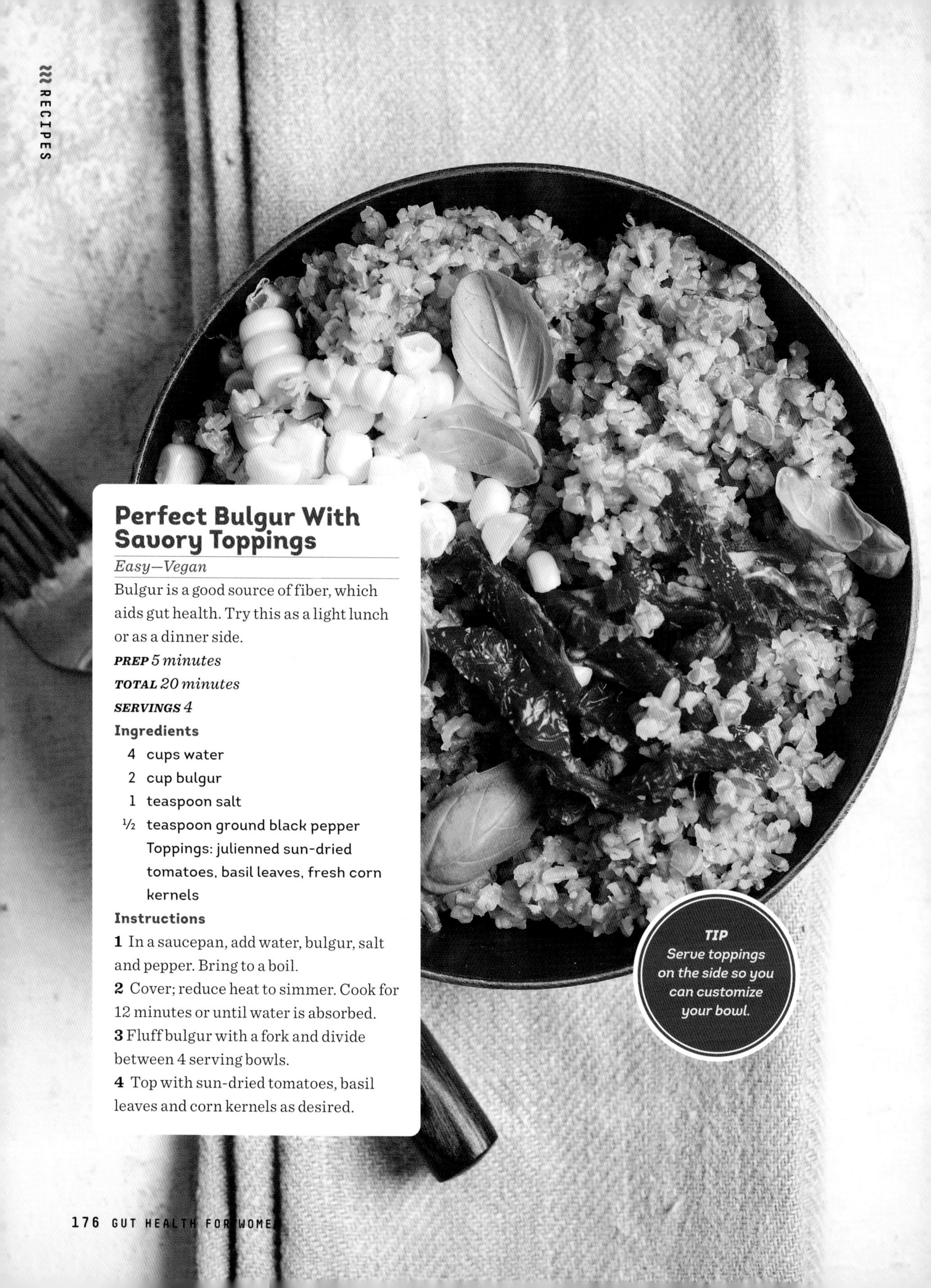

Perfect Bulgur With Savory Toppings

Easy—Vegan

Bulgur is a good source of fiber, which aids gut health. Try this as a light lunch or as a dinner side.

PREP *5 minutes*

TOTAL *20 minutes*

SERVINGS *4*

Ingredients

- 4 cups water
- 2 cup bulgur
- 1 teaspoon salt
- ½ teaspoon ground black pepper
  Toppings: julienned sun-dried tomatoes, basil leaves, fresh corn kernels

Instructions

1 In a saucepan, add water, bulgur, salt and pepper. Bring to a boil.

2 Cover; reduce heat to simmer. Cook for 12 minutes or until water is absorbed.

3 Fluff bulgur with a fork and divide between 4 serving bowls.

4 Top with sun-dried tomatoes, basil leaves and corn kernels as desired.

TIP
Serve toppings on the side so you can customize your bowl.

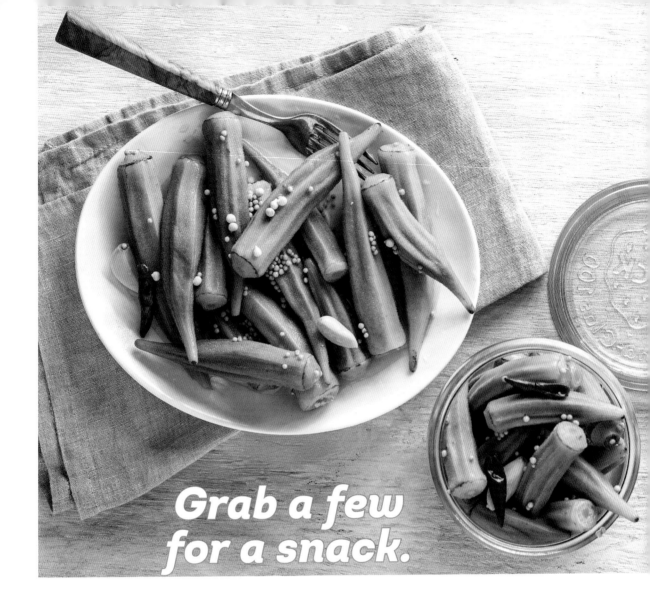

Grab a few for a snack.

Easy Pickled Okra

Gluten Free—Vegan

Enjoy these slightly spicy treats on their own, or serve them as part of a relish tray or cheese board.

PREP *5 minutes*

TOTAL *20 minutes*

SERVINGS *4*

Ingredients

12 whole okra pods

2 whole red cayenne peppers

2 garlic cloves

1½ cups white vinegar

1 tablespoon sea salt

Instructions

1 In a glass pint jar with lid, tightly pack okra. Add peppers and garlic to jar.

2 In a saucepan, bring vinegar and salt to a boil.

3 Reduce heat; simmer for 5 minutes.

4 Slowly pour hot liquid into packed jar.

5 Screw on lid; let cool completely.

6 Refrigerate until ready to serve.

TIP
For a crispy top, caramelize, then let it cool for a minute.

FOR A SWEET END TO ANY MEAL, OR FOR A SNACK ANY TIME, CHECK OUT THESE RECIPES. WE'VE PUT A SPIN ON SOME OF YOUR FAVORITES TO MAKE THEM A BIT GENTLER ON YOUR DIGESTIVE SYSTEM.

Desserts

Crème Brûlée With Mixed Berries

Kid Friendly—Vegetarian

This variation on the classic dessert is much kinder on your gut, because it uses coconut milk instead of cream.

PREP *15 minutes*

TOTAL *1 hour,*
+ 12 hours inactive

SERVINGS *4*

Ingredients

- 2 cups canned coconut milk
- 4 tablespoons honey
- 1 teaspoon salt
- 2 vanilla beans, split and scraped
- 4 egg yolks
- 4 teaspoons maple sugar
- 12 blueberries
- 12 blackberries
- 12 raspberries
- Garnish: mint leaves

Instructions

1 Preheat oven to 300° F.

2 In a saucepan over medium heat, combine coconut milk, honey, salt, seeds from scraped vanilla beans, and vanilla beans. Stir occasionally for 4 minutes, until steam rises, but do not boil. Discard vanilla beans.

3 In a blender, add egg yolks and blend on low for 10 seconds.

4 Slowly pour hot coconut milk mixture through the hole in the lid of the blender.

5 Blend constantly until all milk mixture is incorporated. Go slowly; adding the hot mixture too quickly will scramble the eggs.

6 Slowly pour custard into four 6-ounce ramekins.

7 Place ramekins in a deep baking pan. Pour boiling water into pan until it's about halfway up the sides of the ramekins.

8 Bake 45 minutes. Remove from oven when the custard is slightly firm and a little jiggly in the center.

9 Cool for 1 hour on a wire rack, then cover with plastic wrap and cool overnight in fridge.

10 When ready to serve, sprinkle 1 teaspoon of maple sugar on top of each.

11 Using a kitchen torch (or the broiler of your oven), caramelize the tops.

12 Top with fresh berries and garnish with mint leaves as desired to serve.

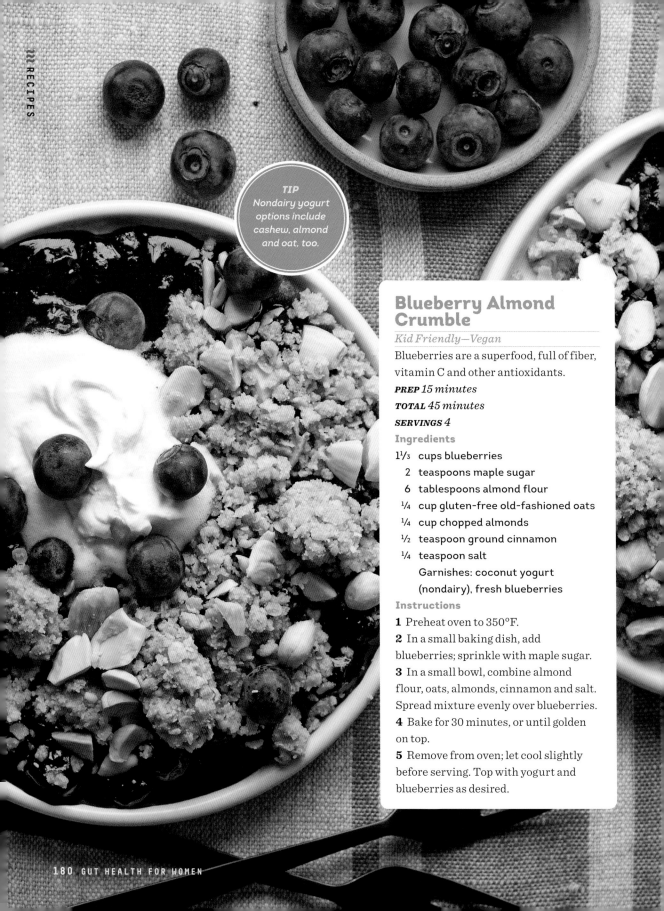

TIP
Nondairy yogurt
options include
cashew, almond
and oat, too.

Blueberry Almond Crumble

Kid Friendly—Vegan

Blueberries are a superfood, full of fiber, vitamin C and other antioxidants.

PREP *15 minutes*

TOTAL *45 minutes*

SERVINGS *4*

Ingredients

1⅓ cups blueberries

2 teaspoons maple sugar

6 tablespoons almond flour

¼ cup gluten-free old-fashioned oats

¼ cup chopped almonds

½ teaspoon ground cinnamon

¼ teaspoon salt

Garnishes: coconut yogurt (nondairy), fresh blueberries

Instructions

1 Preheat oven to 350°F.

2 In a small baking dish, add blueberries; sprinkle with maple sugar.

3 In a small bowl, combine almond flour, oats, almonds, cinnamon and salt. Spread mixture evenly over blueberries.

4 Bake for 30 minutes, or until golden on top.

5 Remove from oven; let cool slightly before serving. Top with yogurt and blueberries as desired.

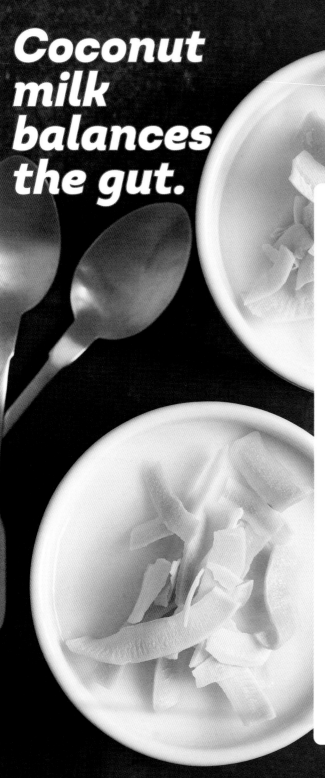

Coconut milk balances the gut.

Toasted Coconut Panna Cotta

Gluten Free—Kid Friendly

Gelatin is good for your skin, bones, hair and gut health.

PREP *25 minutes*

TOTAL *25 minutes, + 12 hours inactive*

SERVINGS *4*

Ingredients

- 4 cups coconut milk, divided
- 1 (¼-ounce) envelope gelatin
- ⅓ cup honey
- 2 teaspoons vanilla
- Garnish: toasted coconut flakes

Instructions

1 In a small saucepan, pour 1 cup coconut milk; sprinkle evenly with gelatin. Let sit for 10 minutes to allow gelatin to soften.

2 Heat milk and gelatin over medium heat, stirring constantly, until gelatin is dissolved.

3 Stir remaining coconut milk and honey into the warm milk. Whisk until dissolved.

4 Remove from heat; stir in vanilla.

5 Let cool for 10 minutes and pour into 4 serving bowls.

6 Cover with plastic wrap and refrigerate overnight.

7 When ready to serve, garnish with toasted coconut flakes.

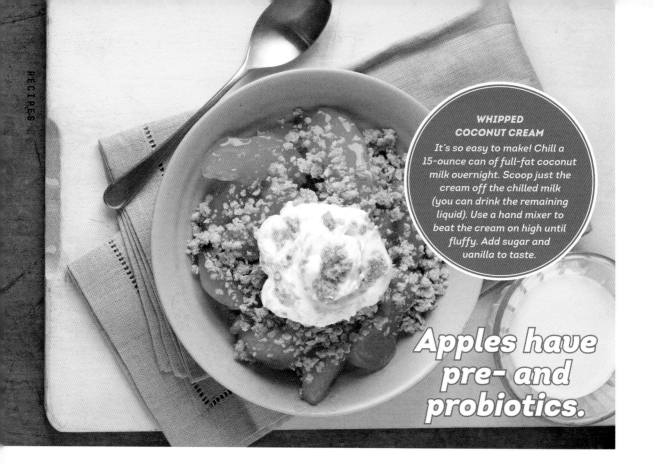

WHIPPED COCONUT CREAM
It's so easy to make! Chill a 15-ounce can of full-fat coconut milk overnight. Scoop just the cream off the chilled milk (you can drink the remaining liquid). Use a hand mixer to beat the cream on high until fluffy. Add sugar and vanilla to taste.

Apples have pre- and probiotics.

Apple Crisp With Coconut Cream

Gluten Free—Kid Friendly—Vegan

Whipped coconut cream keeps this crowd-pleasing dessert vegan—and oh-so-delicious!

PREP *10 minutes*

TOTAL *55 minutes, + 20 minutes inactive*

SERVINGS *4*

Ingredients

Vegetable oil cooking spray

⅓ cup gluten-free almond flour

½ cup gluten-free old-fashioned oats

⅓ cup dark brown sugar

¾ teaspoon cinnamon, divided

⅛ teaspoon salt

¼ cup coconut oil

4 Granny Smith apples, peeled, cored and sliced

⅓ cup maple syrup

½ teaspoon ground cinnamon

⅛ teaspoon nutmeg

Whipped coconut cream

Instructions

1 Preheat oven to 350°F. Grease an 8-inch-square baking pan with vegetable spray.

2 In a large bowl, combine flour, oats, brown sugar, ¼ teaspoon cinnamon, salt and coconut oil.

3 In another large bowl, toss apple slices, maple syrup, remaining cinnamon and nutmeg. Allow to sit for 10 minutes.

4 Place apple mixture in pan; sprinkle oat mixture evenly over the top.

5 Place pan on a baking sheet and bake for 45 minutes, or until topping is light golden brown and filling is bubbling.

6 Remove from oven; cool on wire rack for 10 minutes.

7 Serve warm with whipped coconut cream.

Chocolate Pudding With Cacao Nibs

Easy—Kid Friendly—Vegan

This is a super-healthy dessert or snack option, thanks to chia seeds, protein powder and dark cocoa. Cocoa and cacao nibs are naturally low in sugar, and maple syrup won't cause blood sugar to spike, so #guiltfree!

PREP *5 minutes*

TOTAL *5 minutes, + 1 hour inactive*

SERVINGS *4*

Ingredients

- 2 cups unsweetened almond milk
- 6 tablespoons chia seeds
- ½ cup vegan chocolate protein powder
- ¼ cup dark cocoa powder
- ¼ cup maple syrup
  Garnishes: whipped coconut cream, cacao nibs

Instructions

1 In a blender, mix first 5 ingredients on high for 30 seconds.

2 Pour into 4 serving bowls; refrigerate for 1 hour. Garnish as desired and serve.

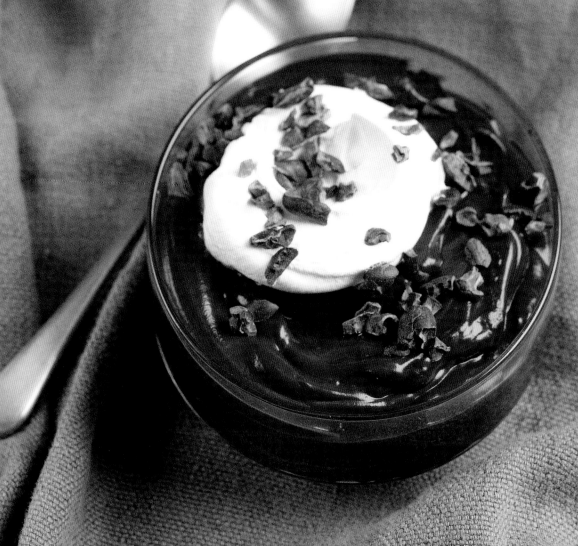

BY THE
Numbers

FROM MOUTH TO FARTHER SOUTH,
YOUR GI TRACT POSTS IMPRESSIVE STATS.

1,000
Number of nutrient-absorbing microvilli on each epithelial cell in the small intestine

4
Hours it takes for the stomach to empty

2
Hours it takes food to move through the small intestine

2
Percentage of an average person's body weight that is bacteria

5 ft.

Length of the large intestine

1 in 100

Proportion of people with celiac disease, an intolerance to gluten, a protein in certain grains

95

Percentage of serotonin in the body that resides in the gut

12 to 24

Hours it takes food to move through the large intestine

22

Number of muscle groups involved in the act of swallowing

20 ft.

Length of the small intestine

25

Percentage of your daily fiber intake that should come from soluble fiber

70

Percentage of the body's immune system that resides in the gut

500 ml.

Volume of gas expelled daily

100 trillion

Number of bacteria thriving in the gut

Fish
    fatty, 141
    which to eat/avoid, 83
Fitness apps, 125
Flavonoids, 64–67
FODMAPs diet, 94, 96, 98–105
Food allergens, 31
Food diary, 71, 96
Food/Foods. *See also* Healthy eating; Recipes
    for better digestion, 84–91
    common, polyphenols in, 67
    fermented. *See* Fermented foods; *specific foods*
    in FODMAPs diet, 104–105
    for a gut reset, 82–83
    for kitchen pantry, 78
    as medicine, 49
    promoting sleep, 141
Food pyramid, mental health, 39
Food triggers, identifying, 82, 101, 103, 148
Fructose, 101
Fruits
    as fiber source, 117
    in FODMAPs diet, 104
    which to eat/avoid, 82

G
Gallbladder, role of, 14
Gamma-Aminobutyric acid (GABA), 140
GAPS (Gut and Psychology Syndrome) diet, 96–97, 147, 148
Gas and bloating
    carbohydrates and, 96, 101
    eliminating. *See* FODMAPs diet
    foods causing, 61, 90
    prebiotics and, 62
    probiotics for, 54
    stress and, 128
Gastrin, 12
Gastrointestinal (GI) tract. *See also* Large intestine; Small intestine; Stomach
    healthy, "clean" diet for, 33
    negative influences on, 9
    statistics on, 184–185
    wall layers, 15
Ginger, 72
Glo (app), 125
Glucose metabolism, 56
L-Glutamine, 72, 87
Gluten-free diets, 62, 96
Grain bowls (recipes), 158–161
Grains
    in FODMAPs diet, 105
    which to eat/avoid, 83
"Green light" food examples, 82–83
Gut-associated lymphoid tissue (GALT), 28
Gut–brain connection, 34–41
Gut–stress connection, 47

H
Headaches, 93, 149
Healthy eating, 76–83
    choosing foods for, 82–83
    pantry items for, 78
    step-by-step plan for, 80–81
Heartburn, cause of, 12
Hepatocytes, 14
Herbal teas, 89
High-FODMAPs diet
    foods in, 104–105
    research findings, 102
Hippocrates, 49
Honey, 86
Human Microbiome Project, 39
Hydration, 111
Hypothalamic-pituitary-adrenal (HPA) axis, 128

I
Immune response triggers, 28, 31, 41
Immune system
    "clean" diet for, 33
    food bolstering, 30
    gut health and, 28
Inflammation, in gut, 27–28
    compromised microbiome and, 31, 33
    foods promoting, 31
    leaky gut and, 28
    signs of, 29
Inflammatory bowel disease (IBD), 44–45
Insulin resistance, 21, 33, 71
Insulin sensitivity, 56, 120
International Human Microbiome Consortium (IHMC), 20
Intestines. *See* Large intestine; Small intestine
Inulin, 87
Irritable bowel syndrome (IBS), 38, 44, 45
    low-FODMAPs diet for, 101, 102
    probiotics and, 54
    serotonin and, 13
    stress-management techniques for, 47

J
Jicama, 87
Jojoba oil, 137

K
Kefir, 33, 56, 82, 88, 120, 137, 141
Keto diet, 62, 81, 96, 102
Kimchi, 5, 33, 56, 88, 120, 140
    recipes, 155, 158, 174
Kira Stokes Fit (app), 125
Kiwi fruit, 141
Kombucha, 51, 53, 56, 87, 120

L
L-Glutamine, 72, 87
Lactobacillus sp., 13, 109, 137

DISCLAIMER Information in *Gut Health for Women* is provided for awareness and education. The benefits and efficacy of various treatments presented in the book are the opinion of the author based on evolving research, anecdotal evidence and expert interviews. There may be differing views on many of the subjects covered. This book is meant to inform and is not a substitute for medical advice and treatment by a licensed physician who knows your complete medical situation, including your history, current signs and symptoms and treatments, including prescription medications. The information herein does not supersede medical advice. Please consult a doctor if you have chronic ailments and/or unresolved health complaints. Results that work for one individual may not work for others. Specific supplement recommendations and advice given herein may not be appropriate for your situation, especially if you have sensitivities, allergies or compromised health. Changing a current treatment may cause symptoms to worsen or lead to unintended side effects. Talk with your doctor before making any changes.

SPECIAL THANKS TO CONTRIBUTING WRITERS:

NANCY COULTER-PARKER, MARGARET MONROE,
JOY PIERCE, BRITTANY RISHER, KATHERINE SCHREIBER,
CARLEY SMITH, KATHRYN DRURY WAGNER

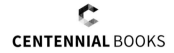

CENTENNIAL BOOKS

An Imprint of
Centennial Media, LLC
40 Worth St., 10th Floor
New York, NY 10013, U.S.A.

ISBN 978-1-951274-21-4

Distributed by
Simon & Schuster, Inc.
1230 Avenue of the Americas
New York, NY 10020, U.S.A.

For information about custom editions, special sales and premium and corporate purchases, please contact Centennial Media at contact@centennialmedia.com.

Manufactured in China

Publishers & Co-Founders Ben Harris, Sebastian Raatz
Editorial Director Annabel Vered
Creative Director Jessica Power
Executive Editor Janet Giovanelli
Deputy Editors Ron Kelly, Alyssa Shaffer
Design Director Ben Margherita
Art Directors Andrea Lukeman,
Natali Suasnavas, Joseph Ulatowski
Assistant Art Director Jaclyn Loney
Photo Editor Christina Creutz
Production Manager Paul Rodina
Production Assistant Alyssa Swiderski
Editorial Assistant Tiana Schippa
Sales & Marketing Jeremy Nurnberg